Penguin Handbooks
The Every Other Day Exercise Book

Fern Lebo is a registered physical and occupational
therapist. She also teaches childbirth education classes
and lectures frequently on 'The Fitness Myth'. She lives
in Toronto with her husband and children.

Fern Lebo

The Every Other Day
Exercise Book

The Easy-Does-It Programme
for Better Bodies

Penguin Books

Penguin Books Ltd, Harmondsworth,
Middlesex, England
Penguin Books, 625 Madison Avenue,
New York, New York 10022, U.S.A.
Penguin Books Australia Ltd, Ringwood,
Victoria, Australia
Penguin Books Canada Ltd, 2801 John Street,
Markham, Ontario, Canada L3R 1B4
Penguin Books (N.Z.) Ltd, 182–190 Wairau Road,
Auckland 10, New Zealand

First published in Canada under the title
The Fitness Myth: A New Approach to Exercise by
Lester and Orpen Limited 1974
Published in Canada under the title *The Every Other Day
Exercise Book: The Easy-Does-It Program for Better Bodies* by
Lester and Orpen Limited 1977
The Every Other Day Exercise Book first published
in the United States of America by
Stein and Day/Publishers 1977
First published in Great Britain by Penguin Books 1979
Published in Penguin Books in the
United States of America 1979

Made and printed in Great Britain by
Hazell Watson & Viney Ltd, Aylesbury, Bucks
Set in Linotype Juliana

To a very special family . . . mine

Contents

Foreword

The Every Other Day Exercise Book is more than just another exercise book. Dealing primarily with 'the normal person', it is an exceptionally complete, accurate, and up to the minute presentation of the essentials required for the maintenance of physical fitness.

In our society, in which the soft sell has been able to make us acquire everything which we need or do not need, it is encouraging to learn from *The Every Other Day Exercise Book* that we do not need to join expensive organizations, and acquire costly apparatus, in order to maintain and promote our own sense of well-being. We have all the necessary equipment in our homes to bring about good muscle tone. All we need do is act.

In our lifetime greater advances have probably taken place in technology than in all prior history. However, these advances have generally resulted in a lessening of physical fitness. *The Every Other Day Exercise Book* enables us, through a simple, but effective means, to learn how to compensate for the loss of muscle tone that has resulted from most of these scientific advances.

Mrs Lebo states, 'Remember that you have a doctor in whom you have confidence and trust; don't hesitate to use him.' This kind of relationship pervades the entire book, thus making of it a meaningful text for the practising physician. Most doctors today do not find the time to sit with their patients and describe the information which is so readily obtained in *The Every Other Day Exercise Book*. I cannot help but conclude that it will become a necessary part of the library of all physicians with a concern for prevention.

The chapters dealing with pregnancy are a real service to all expectant mothers, anticipating fathers, and their obstetricians. Good muscle tone, proper methods of relaxation, can convert 'labour' to the 'joy of having children'.

Brief reference is made to the 'other than normal person' – the heart patient. This serves as a reminder to 'cardiacs' that they can become very fit. It only takes consultation with your doctor, and an appropriate exercise programme.

The Every Other Day Exercise Book communicates knowledge that is essential, in a manner that is simple to comprehend. This unusual text makes compliance a sport. All who use this book will benefit greatly.

N. N. Levinne, M.D., F.C.F.P.
Associate Professor, Family and Community Medicine, University of Toronto.
Director, Family Practice Unit, Mount Sinai Hospital.

Introduction:
Fitness is in Fashion

Introduction

The time has come to take an 'in depth' look at the most popular conversational *hors d'œuvre* on the cocktail circuit: the race for fitness. Fitness fever is infecting ever increasing numbers, and the sharing of health secrets over a glass of Dubonnet has all but replaced the classic toast. Fitness is in fashion. The rising young executive makes some of his or her best contacts on the tennis courts. Major corporate decisions are being made in the saunas, and women, too, eager for that youthful trim, are joining and enjoying the fun of sharing a callisthenics class.

We are being urgently bombarded by every facet of the media to do our bit to get in shape and look naturally beautiful. And of course we all want to. But someone has to trumpet a warning ... take it easy ... be careful ... do it right !

It seems appropriate at this time, even essential, to examine exactly what we mean when we attempt to join the race. Most doctors would explain fitness as the cardiovascular response to exercise. That is, how hard your heart and lungs must work when called upon to perform a specific task.

To most people, fitness means shaping up and slimming down. Looking better. Having the kind of body you've been longing for, one that appears trim and healthy. It becomes obvious then, that the term 'fitness' has different meanings to different people. It is in fact, a little fuzzy. For our purposes however, let us consider it as being in the kind of shape which allows us to function at maximum level with minimum effort, and at the same time, look trim through figure improvement.

When you get started you will discover that fitness can be fun. And more than that, it is also the easiest way we know to live a healthier, more rewarding, perhaps even longer life.

And believe it ! Getting fit is really easy if you know what you're about. But you must know what you are doing in order to achieve your goal without undue risk. Exercise can be potent and should be prescribed for you the same as any other potent prescription ! That's the reason for this book. Exercising made easy !

So what do you do then ? You've decided the time has come to exercise. You may not know the motivating factors behind your decision. Possibly your doctor suggested it. Perhaps you've been reading about the pathetically poor condition of most people. Maybe you've examined your profile and find it's a little too prolific. It could be that the flab is starting to clog up your zipper, or that you tire too easily. Or you've noticed your bottom has a little more bustle than is fashionable. Or you have a nagging ache in the low back region. You could have lost weight from that fantastic diet, but now you've got more skin than you know what to do with. Then too, you may not be able to face a diet but still want to look like you've lost ten years.

Or maybe you're just in lousy shape !

Whatever your reasons, fitness is in fashion. Great news ! But let's be sure you are not one of those unfortunate people who are also hurting themselves while participating in allegedly 'healthy' activities. Let's not have you become one of those statistics. *You* are going to get in shape the sensible way. That means you're about to embark on a programme that's suitable, realistic, and safe for you. A programme designed to fit your needs, for a time you can tolerate, and the freedom to do those exercises you like, and to hell with the ones you don't. Sensibly means knowing a little bit about your anatomy so that you understand the damage one can do by exercising indiscriminately. It also means choosing only those exercises which are inherently safe because of a prior knowledge of body mechanics and basic physiology. And you know? It may be a life saver !

When was the last time you bent down to touch your toes? When you were twelve, I hope ! I can think of no reason why any human being would want to bend down and touch his toes, unless he has a peculiar way of entertaining himself. That's not to say that you may not want to be able to touch your toes – for their own sake : like Mallory's mountain, they're there. But thinking you have to bend down to touch them is part of the fitness myth that millions of people accept as gospel truth.

The fact is that numerous currently accepted exercises for fitness will *not* make you fit. Nor are they designed with your individual safety in mind; they may actually do you harm.

Most people who decide to embark on fitness programmes assume that the people in charge of health clubs, slimming salons, and exercise clinics are experts in their field. In truth, very few of them are. It might shock you to learn that many of these instructors – these executives of exercise – have had a mere six-week course in salesmanship. They lead you to believe that they have some legitimate knowledge of the product they promote – health ! The fact is, you may find your health not improved by their costly merchandise; you may even be hurt in the process.

Of course, there *are* some fitness institutes set up and run scientifically by truly knowledgeable people in the field of exercise. Unfortunately, it has been my experience that these are in the minority. In most cases I have found that the instructors' only qualifications are an attractive physical appearance and some instruction in how to run a floor class. With this they presume to demand that you invest with them your most precious asset – yourself !

It is the false promise of improved health which is my concern, and my reason for writing this book. As a physiotherapist, I have been frequently called upon to treat people with pulled muscles, 'slipped discs', stiff necks, and more: people who simply didn't know how to exercise safely.

A patient of mine, a young man of twenty-seven, had been in a car accident and sustained a severe whiplash. His treatment was long, due to the severity of his injury, but in time the nerve irritation subsided, the pain in his shoulder and arm was relieved, and he had a return of almost full range of movement of his head and neck. After discontinuing his treatment, he decided to join a gym, and was placed in an exercise class. He had the foresight to explain his past history to the instructor, but was assured that he was capable of performing the class exercises. He is back in a cervical collar now; physiotherapy treatments of necessity have been resumed.

The point is, when you begin an exercise class, or when you decide to follow an exercise programme in a magazine or book, the instructor or the author assumes that you are already in top physical condition, that you have no predisposing factors to injury, that the aging processes of your bones and tissues are negligible, and that you can perform the required exercises without harm. Unfortunately, you are in no position to know that this is so until, too often, it is too late. The myth is that you will achieve physical fitness by following an arbitrarily designed exercise programme. It is simply not true.

Most exercises can have safety precautions built right into them in order to avoid undue strain and injury. But it requires a complete knowledge of anatomy and of the physical dynamics of exercise to design these safe exercises. In my experience, I haven't found this to be the case in most of the exercise programmes I have examined. Some exercises should be outlawed for anyone over the age of twenty-one because of the risk involved in performing them, yet they appear with alarming regularity in articles, books, and exercise club programmes. Alternative exercises which avoid undue risk and still achieve the desired favourable results are conspicuously absent from nearly every exercise sheet I have examined in the course of my research.

Many exercise clubs now request a certificate of good health from your doctor before they allow you to begin their exercise programmes. That signature may help them to avoid a costly law suit, but it may not help you to avoid injury. Even when your doctor tells you to go ahead and exercise for the good of your health, unless he is a specialist in the field of exercise, he really is not equipped to know which exercises are safe for you and which are not.

I have visited some of these 'health havens' and met the mini-skirted young ladies who escort you gently through the luxurious facilities. I have met their pitch-men, those fast-talking salesmen who spin incredible tales about melting fat through friction and other such nonsense, the men who promise that merely by signing on the dotted line, and investing a small fortune, you can achieve miracles. Their vast array of equipment is tempting; their atmosphere is relaxing; you may feel that coming to such a place will improve your incentive. But be aware that you may be as much of an expert as anyone else in the place!

I think that you can accomplish your aim at home, without the benefit of costly frills, but if you are the type who requires company for motivation, then search out an authentic fitness institute. Here are a few simple questions you will want answered before you decide on a place.

Is there a doctor on call at all times?
Is resuscitation equipment available on the spot?
Will you be monitored, and put through a series of stress tests, before beginning the programme?
Is your programme individually designed for you by a qualified person with suitable medical background?
Will you progress on the basis of physical tests performed under monitored conditions?

If all the answers to the above questions are in the affirmative, you have most likely found yourself a reliable fitness place.

I would like to dispel a few more fitness fairy tales being sold at fantastic prices to unsuspecting heavies desperate to lose weight. Exercise alone will not take the pounds off. That's fact! The amount of exercise required to use up enough calories to produce a weight loss is phenomenal and highly unrealistic. Dieting is the *only* way to lose poundage. But dieting alone does not achieve the result of dieting *and* exercise. Exercise tones and tightens your muscles so that as you lose weight, you become firmer and tighter in those areas where you need it. Exercise alone can reduce your measurements by redistributing your weight, so that you may lose a size without losing weight – which may be all that you need to do. So don't be misled by the promise of a great weight loss just by signing a contract which allows you so many hours of 'easy' exercises.

Some body boutiques feature unusual techniques and gimmicks, such as wrapping you up mummy-like, turning on the heat, and presenting you with an undeniable weight loss when it's all over. The problem is that the scale merely shows you how much fluid you have lost – how much you have perspired. Drinking any liquid will replace that weight loss in a matter of hours, and you're right back where you started.

Most of these same salons advise you to cut down on your fluid intake while receiving treatments. You may do so if you wish, but it isn't healthy! After all, it isn't fluid that makes you fat, it's fat. If you are truly losing weight, your fluid intake will have little to do with it, and daily quantities of fluid are essential to the maintenance of normal good health. If you *are* one of the few people who retain fluids in abnormally high amounts, enough to make you swell and appear heavier than you actually are, you are in need of a qualified physician. He may want you to begin using specific medication or a suitably adjusted and restricted diet. Obviously this is not the sort of thing for the layman to decide.

I feel compelled to say a few words about yoga, an ancient art originating in India, and more recently, a craze which has been the 'in' thing for many people of the Western world. I have no doubt that if started early enough, and followed religiously, it provides great benefits in physical and mental well being, as is true of any continuous exercise regime. However, I have seen many middle-aged men and women desperately seeking the relief of a physiotherapist's department as the result of attempting to imitate some lovely yogini on television, or even after what was designed to be an individually adapted class. A woman of fifty-five, attending such a class, was complimented on her youthful agility, and, encouraged to twist just a little bit more, tore some small ligaments in her back. Her case, unfortunately, is not rare enough.

Some of the postures which require great twisting or hyperextension of the lower back can have serious consequences if one should have any of the degenerative disc changes common to middle age, or even if one has neglected a regular exercise routine over a period of years. Straining beyond one's capacity is simply imprudent and absurd, and that is what some of the movement in yoga may do.

Another balloon I'd like to pop is the one that promises

that the machines will do it all for you. They can't – it's as simple as that! If the machine is exercising, most likely you are not. If the machine is easy enough for a child to manoeuvre, it's too easy for you. Some machines are even reputed to 'break up the fat'. Physiologically, it doesn't work that way. No matter how much you're bounced around, if you've got fat, you've still got it, and maybe a few bruises as a bonus.

A patient of mine bought an expensive exercise chair, with the promise that the pounds would fall off as she watched television. Unfortunately, although she didn't know it at the time, she had the beginnings of a degenerative disc, very common for her age. The result was no weight loss, but a 'slipped disc' for which she is now receiving treatment.

The average muscle if not used sufficiently loses its tone. This means that the individual muscle fibres lose their resiliency and spring. As you exercise them, these fibres plump up and take up the slack. In order to regain resilience you must work your muscles against increasing resistance. Unless the machine is providing you with real resistance to work against, it is providing you with nothing.

All of this is not really new. Any physiotherapist, and most doctors, can verify it, and perhaps add a little more. But they are not in the practice of advertising; as a result, most people are falsely led to believe that the 'fat factories' are the only way to fitness. The fact is, you can arrange a better exercise programme yourself, one that is safe, easy, and effective.

Part One of this book consists of general exercises which provide in themselves the increasing resistance you require, so that you improve as you work. These exercises deal with all parts of the body. They are arranged so that you can choose appropriate exercises yourself for a programme that is medically sound. By selecting just three or four exercises from each chapter that involves your specific trouble area, you design a routine to fit your own individual needs and life style. All the exercises included are safe for the average person to do, although you may still want to check them out with your doctor if you have previously suffered from a medically diagnosed condition. They are also easy to understand, and most do not need explanatory drawings: I have included these only where necessary.

In some cases, I have not mentioned an exact number of times to perform a specific exercise. It is understood that you will begin with the number of times that is comfortable for you, and progress at your own rate. *There is no maximum number of times that any exercise should be done*: halt the progression when you feel fit, and use that final number for maintenance of tone in the area you have been working on.

If, however, you wish to do a maintenance programme for the entire body, you will find all you require in Part Two of this book: Sixteen Minutes to Keep Your Shape. There, in a simple sixteen-minute programme, are all the components necessary for general maintenance plus the development of cardiovascular and respiratory fitness. It is a super programme and following it every other day will surely put you in tip-top condition all over.

Remember that exercising requires extra work on the part of your entire body system, so it is a good idea not to exercise immediately before a large meal, or for an hour or so afterwards. Remember, too, that strenuous exercising produces sweat, so give yourself a few minutes, after completing your programme, to cool down without becoming chilled.

I was asked, during the writing of this book, to include chapters for arthritics and for people suffering from medically-diagnosed back injuries. However, each would really require a book of its own. Aside from the obvious limitations of space, I could not in all conscience do so. Arthritis is a disease which encompasses so many variables that a myriad of text-books have been written on the subject.

Back injuries are another complicated story. Low back pain is one of the most common complaints met by the physio-therapist. Its causes are diverse; a doctor may find that it is due to disease of the kidneys or pancreas, a malignancy of bone or bowel, prostatitis, or a host of varying spinal prob-lems. When considering spinal abnormalities which may be causing the pain, the situation is further obscured by the psy-chological aspect which intrudes with many patients. It has also been learned that intervertebral disc protrusions, which commonly cause sciatic pain, *can* give rise to low back pain without sciatica.

When treating a patient with low back pain of a serious nature, success is based on careful consideration of the indi-vidual patient, and his condition as a whole. 'It involves not only the temporary relief of pain, but also, removal of the underlying cause to prevent recurrence.'[1]

One cannot generalize when it comes to diseased tissue; as a physiotherapist, I know how dangerous the results can be. This book is concerned, then, not with disease, convalescence, or rehabilitation, but with the average person who is in poor condition and wants to be fit.

Part Three: Pre-natal Care deals not only with fitness in the general sense, but also with the body changes of preg-nancy and the effects of these changes. Here I talk about total life style during pregnancy, a topic which has been a specialty of mine for many years. Often I have had expectant mothers come to me not only for guidance in keeping fit, but also for help in understanding the physiological changes of pregnancy and how to enjoy safely the months ahead. In this chapter I hope to answer many of these questions.

1. Philip Wiles. *Essentials of Orthopedics* (Baltimore: Williams and Wilkins, 1965).

There are differences of opinion even among members of the medical profession as to the value of an exercise programme in post-cardiac care. In Part Four I have presented a reasonable case for a safe approach to exercise based upon current medical research.

Part One:
Your Choice

1 Basic Back Care

Let's talk about basic anatomy.

Your back consists of the vertebral column, or spine, and the soft structures relating to it. The spine provides the back with both stability and mobility. For stability it is dependent on the large muscles, ligaments, discs, normal curvatures, and bony joints. For mobility it depends on the elasticity of ligaments, the compressibility and elasticity of the discs, and the relative positions of the bony joints. The interrelationship of these structures, and their interdependability, form a complex entity.

The muscles of the back, for the most part, are very small, and span no more than two or three inches in length. These muscles, attached along the back of the vertebral column, help prevent too much flexion, or forward-bending of the spine. Conversely, the abdominal muscles, although not directly attached to the structures of the back, help prevent too much extension of the spine by providing a counterbalancing effect, and therefore play a vital role in back care. That is often why the unlucky man with a protuberant pot belly and weakened abdominal muscles usually suffers from a low back ache.

The discs between the vertebrae act as buffers, a necessity in walking or jumping. They help to reduce strain on the bony structures by absorbing shock. But it is important to note that these discs become avascular after the age of twenty-one. That is, they lose their blood supply, and it follows that there is a subsequent loss of water and 'sponginess', and so of the ability to absorb shock. Degenerative disc changes are then obviously not limited to the aged. An awareness of that fact is important for the safe performance of exercises.

If all this anatomy sounds complicated and dull, just remember that when all these structures work well together they accomplish their one main function in life – they help you to stand erect. Usually they do that rather well. Occasionally, however, like a bolt from the blue comes sudden and extremely painful back pain. It may occur after an unusual movement, or a movement of stress such as rotation, or bending down with knees straight. Sometimes the pain does not begin for a day or two, but when it does, it can be severe enough to warrant a physician's attention, and, frequently, follow-up physiotherapy treatments.

Maybe you're one of the unfortunate thousands who suffer from a miserable aching in the low back area. It could be chronic back strain, due simply to poor posture, aging processes, or the residual effects of a previous injury.

Even if right now you are lucky enough not to suffer from any back complaint, it's easy to become a member of this not-so-elite clan if you neglect proper care and safety. It's this lack of common sense which so irritates me when I watch an allegedly well-run callisthenics class which demands twisting, torsion, and toe touching, and demonstrates an obvious ignorance of the basic aspects of back welfare on the part of the instructor.

The small muscles and ligaments of the back were not meant for weight-lifting – certainly not for lifting more than half your own body weight against the resistance of gravity. That is precisely what you ask them to do every time you bend down to touch your toes. They don't like you for that, and may go into spasm in spite! That is what strained muscles usually do in order to protect themselves from further strain. Muscle spasm and pain work as defence mechanisms of the body and must not be ignored.

Should you unknowingly or suddenly perform a movement beyond the elastic capabilities of your muscles or ligaments, they may actually tear, thus allowing for more serious injury to other soft structures of the back. This is the real danger of exercising along with your favourite television personality.

What does all this have to do with your exercise programme? Well, unless you have a written guarantee that your back is in A-1 fail-safe condition, stooping is out. That includes all exercises which involve bending down with straight knees and touching your toes. If you want to limber up, there are safer and more effective ways to do it. Most of us over twenty-one don't know if we have a weakness in our back until unexpectedly we 'throw it out'. Do yourself a favour – save it!

Something I've mentioned only briefly is that every back should have a normal amount of curvature. That is, the upper

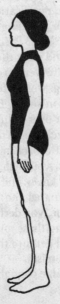

part curves, or bows out slightly, while the lower part curves in a bit. The little muscles in front and back of the spine help to maintain this normal curve. But when muscles are strained, they usually react by going into spasm – that is, shortening their length, which serves to increase or accentuate that normal curvature. And that produces dull aching, perhaps even sharp pain.

The best way to relieve muscle spasm is to stretch it out. The muscles then respond by relaxing; they have no choice. A good old-fashioned massage may sound good – it may even feel good – but it takes too long. Instead, just put a gentle continuous stretch on those muscles and you've got fast relief. It's a physiological phenomenon, and it's easy to do. Bend one knee towards your chest and you automatically flatten out the low back curve. Needless to say, if one knee is good, two are even better. But that's hard to do while you're standing!

Think of the fantastic ramifications of this new discovery. You're washing dishes or standing at the stove and you put one foot on a low stool. Voilà! You immediately straighten out the low back curve and relax those tired muscles.

Here's another new discovery. You may have seen exercise men on television doing wonderful sit-ups. That's fine for them, they're paid to be in shape. But you may be asking for trouble if you make your over-indulged stomach muscles pull you up; if they are too weak to do the job without extra help, they call upon your little back muscles to tighten up and stabilize the area, and so your aching back appears. How to avoid that? Bend your knees and come up that way. You have mechanically eliminated the possibility of muscle substitution; at the same time, you derive maximum benefit from the exercise, by only using those muscle groups for which the exercise was designed. I'll get into this more specifically in the chapter on abdominal exercises.

I really cannot emphasize enough how dangerous it can be

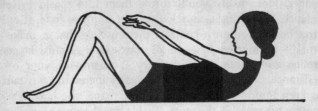

to follow some television exerciser's suggestions on sit-ups, twisting exercises, and double leg lifts. If you're in great shape, and have had the working capacity of your muscles checked recently, you just might be able to handle it. If you haven't, and are relying on chance, you're making a fool's bet. You are simply not in a position to judge whether or not your own muscles are sufficiently strong to perform those exercises safely and without the possibility of unknowingly substituting the wrong muscle groups. It takes an expert to make that judgement. I have seen all too often the results of such foolhardy gambles limping into the physiotherapy department. If you find you need the group feeling while you exercise as a form of personal motivation, why not get together with a few of your friends on a regular basis, choose those exercises in the book which best suit you, and form your own body shop?

Exercising, you see, involves more than just making a few windmills. It involves safety and common sense. It means not asking your muscles to do more than they are capable of doing. It means working to maximum capacity for maximum benefit, and knowing the mechanical tricks to avoid undue strain.

A very common error in exercise is to use momentum to get you where you couldn't get on muscle power alone, and that involves uncontrolled movement. Although you may want to stretch some muscles in the hopes of becoming more limber, more likely you'll throw them into spasm in self-defence. Stretching a muscle does *not* improve tone, it only stretches it. You must contract the muscle – that is, make it work – to improve tone. So all your exercises must be controlled and within your capacity. You provide your own resistance. Since it requires continually increasing resistance to keep improving muscle tone and shape, the harder you work your muscles, the more capable they become of working even harder. Best of all, it's *safe* !

If you think I am placing a great deal of emphasis on looking after your back, you're right ! The most powerful biceps in the world are of little use if you can't get around to show them off. That lithe figure you've been working so hard to achieve is just a distraction if there's a crimp in your walk. If you can't stand tall and move with authority, you're not in good shape no matter how many deep knee bends you can boast. So before you begin your exercise programme, consider your normal everyday activities and how you can make them work for you.

LIFTING Dropped a paper clip? Here's a good chance to use your leg muscles. Bend your knees and down you go with a straight back. Are you lifting a heavy carton? Let your legs lift it for you. You squat, you wrestle with it, then you use your powerful quadriceps – those big muscles in the front of your thighs – to get you on your feet. If you still can't lift it, it's probably too heavy, so get some help. You see how simple it can be? Not only that, it may save you from a long rest flat on your back in bed. Bend your knees; that's their function.

CARRYING You do the shopping and valiantly stagger homeward, bags abreast, back bent like a sapling in the wind. No wonder your little muscles are aching to act up. If you have too much to carry properly, enlist another person, or use a shopping bag on wheels. Do use common sense. Or here's a neat little trick: divide your load so you carry half in each hand in shopping bags, or even clutched in close. You thus lessen the strain on your back, also on your heart. You carry the same load with much less effort.

SAFE AND SOUND Statistics say that you're more likely to take that trip fantastic at home than anywhere else. What can you do to make the odds more reasonable? A small investment at your local hardware store may give you your biggest payoff. How about some safety strips in your bath or shower? That packet could be a life saver.

Be concerned about what you wear on your feet around the house. I have good news: barefoot is healthy! Those five-toed wonders are beautifully designed to give you excellent traction, and when you go barefoot you allow your muscles the freedom to do their work.

A patient of mine, whose habit it was to wear cosy knitted slippers around the house, bought a lovely split-level home, stairs included. Before she'd had a chance to make even the first mortgage payment, those dainty little devils were her downfall. On thickly carpeted steps, they're deadly. A bad fall, a few broken bones, an added mortgage, and she was prepared to take my barefoot advice.

However, if bare feet leave you cold, be sure to look for slippers with a grip.

STANDING If you have to stand on your feet all day, you may be subject to aching feet, cramped legs, sore back. Although I can't provide a cot on the spot for such people, I can suggest a technique to ease the strain. Find a low stool and rest one foot on it. When you do that, you have mechanically straightened out the low back curve and brought

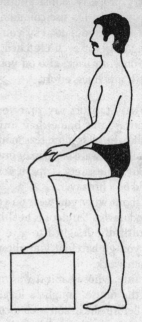

relief to your low back muscles. Alternate your feet, and you find you tire less easily as the strain is decreased. If a stool is inconvenient and you stand at a counter, use the bottom ledge of that counter for the same effect. Walking around helps too, as your leg muscles assist with a pumping action to aid venous return to the heart. And do sit down whenever you don't have to stand.

SLEEPING If you find you are waking in the mornings with low back ache, there are a few techniques you can use while you sleep to help reduce the discomfort. If you like to sleep on your back, a good trick is to place a pillow under your knees.

This serves to tilt the pelvis backward, effectively straightening the low back curve and thus reducing strain.

If you like to sleep on your side, bend at least one knee. A pillow under the upper knee may also be of help.

A good bed is important too. A firm box spring is probably enough, but a length of plywood under the mattress is helpful if you really need it. A soft mattress may feel comfortable when you lie down on it, but it requires too much muscle work for proper relaxation.

Another point to remember is that a foam rubber pillow is harder on your neck muscles than the old-fashioned kind. Foam has recoil and requires muscle use during sleep. A feather or kapok pillow, on the other hand, supports the head and moulds itself to it, allowing muscles in spasm to relax.

2 Posture

If your gym teacher at school taught you to stand up straight, chin up, shoulders back and chest out, she didn't know much about good posture. If you learned how to stand straight in the army, then you know the agony of trying to maintain that ridiculous posture for any length of time.

Posture is the position or attitude of the body in space. There are specific muscles called the antigravity muscles, which work with the maximum efficiency and minimum effort when posture is correct. It follows that poor posture produces unnecessary work for muscles, and causes aches.

If you don't feel that your posture is as good as it might be, you can check it out in front of a mirror. A word of warning: your corrected posture won't feel natural to you at first. You may feel silly or slightly off-balance. After all, you haven't been standing that way all your life, and it feels peculiar. You'll find, however, that as you continue to think consciously of it, and to check yourself often at first, you'll become accustomed to where your body is in space. You will not only feel better, you'll look better. A general exercise routine will also help you towards better posture as your muscles improve in tone and you begin to feel better about your appearance.

What is good normal posture? Stand in front of a mirror and check yourself on the following points:

(1) feet spaced four or five inches apart and toes pointed forward;

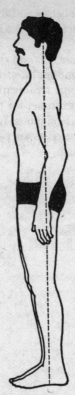

(2) weight distributed evenly, and slightly in front of your ankles; ankle joints at ninety degrees;

(3) knees firm but not locked;

(4) hip joints directly over knee joints;

(5) slight low back curve;

(6) slight upper back curve;

(7) slight neck curve;

(8) head well set on spine so eyes look forward;

(9) shoulders and hips level.

These are nine steps to a better position in life. You may even find you have 'grown' an inch or two in the process.

If you find your posture is far off the norm, let your doctor check for structural abnormalities. If you require, he will send you for physiotherapy treatments. It would be presumptuous of me to include exercises for posture correction without knowing the medical diagnosis. Indeed, it could be harmful. Posture correction exercises are easy and worthwhile, but first consult your physician.

3 Stomach Exercises

That bulge around your belt is probably the first thing you notice when you begin to face the awful reality – you're out of shape! You try to camouflage it by wearing up-and-down stripes, but somehow they take a detour around the fifth button. Maybe you even tighten your belt to kid yourself along, but alas, it all hangs out.

What should you do now that panic has set in? Once you know what's safe for you, you can make good use of the pool and the gym. But *you* decide on the basis of what you've learned; don't leave it in the hands of instructors. I've given more deep heat treatments to ex-callisthenics addicts than I care to count.

And as I mentioned before, forget the machines. No thumping, pummelling, or bumping is going to carve you slim. You have to work your muscles voluntarily in order to shed those unsightly inches.

Now what about abdominal exercises? What can you really do safely to tighten up and trim down? And why bother?

Your abdominals are the large group of muscles in front of your body that flatten your stomach and help you appear trim. They also have the important job of helping to support your internal organs. They may be the least used of all your large muscle groups; if you're fairly inactive, if you have a desk job, and an athletic afternoon means a walk to the coffee machine, you're a prime candidate for the executive hang-over.

With all abdominal exercises comes an added bonus : at the same time that you're pulling in your belt, you are also strengthening the small muscles of the spine. Two for the price of one !

If your abdominal muscles are really weak, you'll know it when you try to hold a position. The muscles will start to tremble and you won't be able to hold the contraction. Just progress slowly until you are able to hold the contraction without trembling. If you haven't got that tremble, you may begin by doing each exercise you choose five times and holding for a count of five. Increase daily, first by increasing the number of times by two each day until you reach twenty-five, then by increasing your count for the hold. Remember to give each muscle contraction your best effort.

Choose three or four exercises and do them conscientiously. If they look easy, it's because they are, but they're also just as effective as any abdominal exercises you may find elsewhere. Since they have built-in safety features, they will not hurt you.

Tip: All exercises should be done on the firmest support available – the floor.

1 PELVIC TILT (so easy you can't afford not to do it)

Lying on your back, bend both knees so that your feet are flat on the floor. Slip your hand under the small of your back and feel a slight hollow. Now press your back down into your hand – that is, flatten your back. Remove your hand and try it again. Repeat and hold the contraction. Relax.

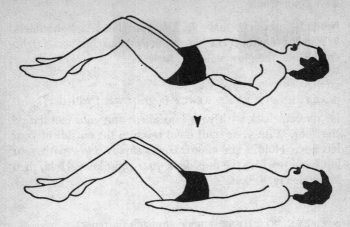

2 KNEE REACH (as effective as a sit-up, but safe)

Lie on your back with your knees bent so your feet are flat on the floor. With both hands reach out to touch your knees or

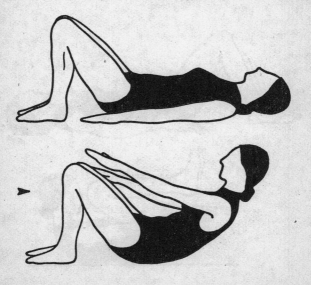

beyond if you can make it. Lift your head and shoulders, keeping your chin tucked in and your stomach muscles tightened. Hold, then lower slowly. Repeat .

3 ALTERNATE KNEE REACH (a great waist whittler)

Lie on your back with your knees bent and your feet flat on the floor. With your right hand reach to the outside of your left knee. Hold it and count. Lower slowly. Now with your left hand reach to the outside of your right knee. Hold, then lower slowly. Repeat.

4 KNEES TO CHEST (a good stomach flattener)

Lie on your back with your knees bent and your feet flat on the floor. Your hands should remain at your sides, palms down, and act as a support only. Tighten your abdominal

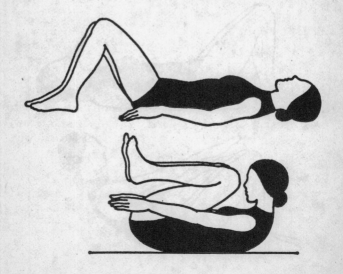

muscles and slowly pull up your knees to your chest. Lower slowly to starting. Repeat. You may progress by combining this movement with the knee reach. Do them together. Hold. Lower slowly. Then repeat.

5 ABDOMINAL BREATHING (a toner and relaxer all in one)

Lie on your back with your legs stretched out. Breathe in slowly through your nose while making your stomach rise. Slowly exhale through your mouth tightening your stomach muscles to get rid of all the air. Do this no more than two or three times in succession, but repeat at intervals throughout your exercise routine.

6 ALTERNATE KNEE TO CHEST (hits you below the belt)

Lie on your back with your knees bent and your feet flat on the floor. Tighten your stomach muscles and pull up one knee to your chest. Hold for the count, then lower slowly. Repeat with other knee. Repeat.

7 ALTERNATE KNEE TO ELBOW (a more advanced version of the knee reach)

Lie on your back with knees bent and feet flat on the floor. Put your hands on your shoulders. With your right elbow, reach to touch your left knee and try to sit up. Lower slowly. With your left elbow, reach to your right knee. Repeat.

8 HUMPING AND HOLLOWING (good for stomach *and* back)

Get on your hands and knees with your hands directly under your shoulders, and your knees directly under your hips.

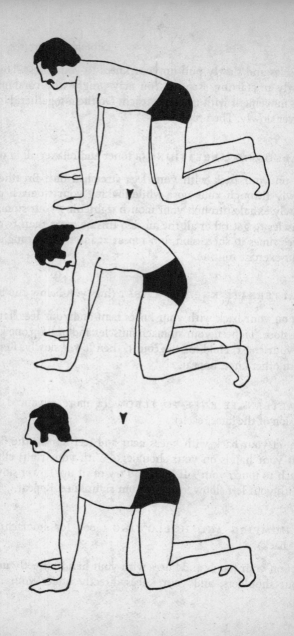

Tighten your abdominals, tuck your head down, and slowly hump your back like a cat. Hold it. Slowly look up, arch your back, and point your posterior up. Repeat.

9 HUMPING AND HOLLOWING WITH A KICK (a progression of 8)

Up on your hands and knees as above. This time, as you hump your back, bring your right knee up to touch your head. As you slowly arch your back, look up towards the ceiling and stretch your right leg behind you. Do this then with your left leg. Repeat.

10 SIT LIFT (strong exercise for abdominals)

Sit on a sturdy chair and grip the seat with your hands. Straighten your legs so that they are out in front of you, and, by pushing up on your hands, lift your entire body off the chair. Hold, relax, repeat.

4 Breathing Exercises

All your life you've been breathing. Maybe by now you consider yourself an expert. You're quite right, of course. For normal quiet respiration, the inhaling of air is the result of muscle contraction. You don't have to think about it; your body looks after it for you. When you've been working hard, or exercising strenuously, you breathe more deeply, and that's automatic as well. It's actually a reflex: there is a rhythmical discharge of impulses from your respiratory centre which is influenced by chemical and nervous factors.

But there are other ways to breathe which you may find very helpful. Deep breathing, done when you are relaxed, can increase your feeling of well-being immeasurably. It increases the amount of oxygen available to the body and is especially helpful during relaxation. You may also be able to increase your lung capacity so that you feel better after exertion – you aren't starved for air.

Tip: Too much oxygen can make you dizzy, so don't do too many deep breaths in succession; three is enough. Space your deep breathing throughout your exercise routine, and make use of it when you are trying to relax.

1 ABDOMINAL BREATHING

Put your hands, palms down, on your stomach. Using your hands to press down, blow out all the air from your lungs.

Then slowly, very slowly, breathe in through your nose making your stomach expand or rise. Breathe out through your mouth, letting your stomach relax.

2 LATERAL COSTAL BREATHING

Put your hands, palms down, on your lower ribs. Using your hands to press down on your ribs, blow out all the air you have in your lungs. Now relax your hands and breathe in slowly through your nose, spreading your rib cage as you do so. As you exhale, relax.

5 Low Back Exercises

I have talked at some length about aching backs, low back discomfort, and how to care for your back during both exercising and everyday activities. I want to make it clear that I am talking about the normal kinds of aches and pains we all experience at some time or other. If, however, you are suffering from severe back pain, either constant or intermittent, that definitely calls for the attention of a qualified physician. You will likely find that he endorses wholeheartedly the exercises found in this book (after all, they are medically sound), but do check with him before beginning a back programme.

If you get the usual run of I'm-tired-and-my-back-hurts aches, then a few good back exercises should be included in your exercise programme. If you want to avoid low back discomfort, then you need back exercises. They will help strengthen the small muscles around the spine, and thus reduce strain by increasing support to the back.

Choose three or four of the following exercises and include them in your routine. Many of them are the same as those included in the chapter on abdominal exercises. That is because, while exercising your back muscles, you invariably include exercise to another large muscle group, the abdominals.

Begin by doing those exercises you choose five times each every day, holding the contraction for a count of five. As that begins to feel too easy, progress by increasing the number of times you do the exercise, until you reach twenty-five, then increase the length of holding.

1 PELVIC TILT (a definite must)

Lying on your back with your knees bent so that your feet
are flat on the floor, slip your hand under the small of your
back. You will feel a slight hollow. Now press your back
down into your hand – that is, flatten your back. Remove
your hand and press down again. Hold and count. Let go,
then repeat.

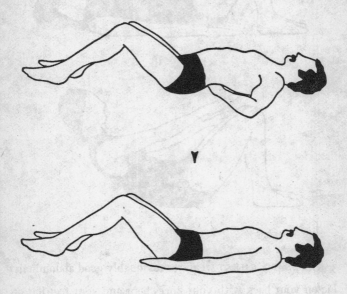

2 KNEE REACH (good for what ails you)

Lie on your back with your knees bent and your feet flat on
the floor. With both hands reach out to touch your knees and
try to sit up. Lift your head and shoulders, keeping your chin

tucked in and tightening your abdominal muscles. Lower yourself slowly. Repeat.

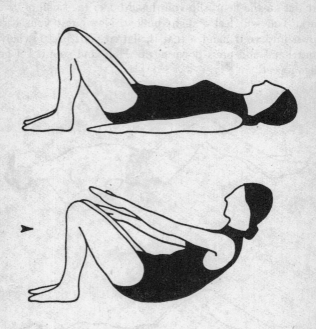

3 KNEES TO CHEST (requires reasonably good abdominals)

Lie on your back with your knees bent and your feet flat on the floor. Keep your hands at your sides, palms down, and use them only for support. Tighten your abdominal muscles and slowly pull up your knees to your chest. Lower slowly to starting position. Repeat. You may progress by combining this exercise with the knee reach. Do them together, hold and relax.

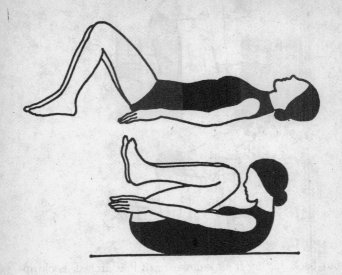

4 HUMPING AND HOLLOWING (great for limbering up the back)

Get up on your hands and knees, with your hands directly under your shoulders and your knees directly under your hips. Tighten your abdominals, tuck your head down, and slowly hump your back like a cat. Hold it. Now slowly relax

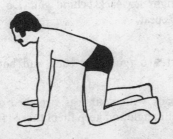

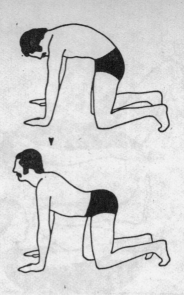

your back, letting it sink down until it is arched. Look up-
wards as you do this, and point your posterior up. Repeat.

5 HUMPING AND HOLLOWING WITH A KICK (a progres-
sion of 4)

Up on your hands and knees as above. This time as you hump
your back, bring your right knee up to touch your head. As
you slowly arch your back, look up towards the ceiling and
stretch your right leg back behind you. Do this then with
your left leg. Repeat.

6 BACK ARCHING (good for back and bottom but very
strenuous)

Lie on your back with your legs stretched out. Bend your
elbows to a right angle and keep them tucked in at your sides.

Tighten hips and back muscles, and slowly arch your back by pushing off at the heels, elbows, and head. Hold. Repeat.

7 BACK STRETCHER (tough but worth the effort)

Lie on your stomach, face down, and clasp your hands behind your head or neck. Raise your head and shoulders, keeping your chin tucked in. Hold. Lower and repeat.

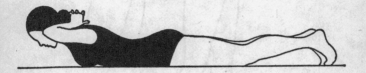

8 THE ROCKER (a progression of 7)

Lie on your stomach with hands clasped behind your head. Tuck your chin in and arch your back by raising your head and shoulders and both legs.

If you are determined to do some back mobility exercises because somewhere in your past you understood that stretching muscles does something magical to them, here are three good exercises. I don't recommend them for anyone with back aches, but if you really want to loosen up, or if you're an athlete, go ahead and try them out.

9 MERRY-GO-ROUND

Stand up straight, space your feet about eighteen inches apart. Place your hands on your hips and lean forward. Slowly

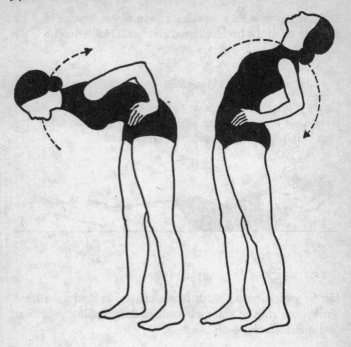

rotate your body from the waist moving clockwise. Feel a good stretch on those muscles. Go around five times and then repeat, going counter-clockwise.

10 STRETCH AND REACH (good for back and legs – if you can make it)

Standing up straight, space your feet about eighteen inches apart. Reach out with both hands so that they are in front of you, and bend forward from the waist. Your back should be

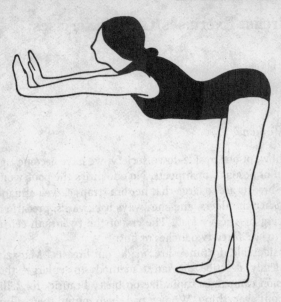

arched, not rounded, and your head lifted so that your eyes point skyward. Now bounce.

11 SIDE WINDER (requires good muscle strength and fair
   courage)

Lie face down with your hands at your sides. Lift your head and shoulders off the floor. Bend your trunk to alternate sides.

6 Breast Exercises/Chest Exercises

For Women

Somehow, in our upside-down society, we have become a generation of bosom worshippers. No one pities the poor woman whose breasts are so large that her bra straps carve permanent ruts in her shoulders, and she sways backwards, precariously balancing her heavy load. The cry of the twentieth century seems to be: forty-two inches or bust!

Considerable fortunes are made on breasts. Magazines breathlessly describe the latest methods to 'enlarge' them. Television campaigns capitalize on busty beauties for selling just about everything. Women pad them, pump them, plump them, inject them, balloon them, festoon them – all because they believe that the bosom somehow is the epitome of sexiness.

Breast tissue, however, is not muscle tissue, even though the advertisements for breast enlargers might have you believe otherwise. Breasts are actually composed mostly of fatty tissue and glandular tissue. That means there is nothing you can do to change their size, no matter what the hormone cream ads promise. That means that if you are over endowed, nothing short of reduction surgery, or a strenuous diet to lose some of the extra fat, is going to make you a fashionable flatty. It also means that if you think your breasts are embarrassingly tiny, you simply *cannot* change their size with weights, pulleys, or massage. When you exercise madly at your health club, and congratulate yourself on having increased your measurements by three-quarters of an inch, what you have actually succeeded in doing is increasing the musculature of your back. If all you want is a bigger bra size, then do try the back exercises – but beware the connoisseur of the cup !

What about the natural look? Those liberated ladies who scorn all encumbrances designed by men to restrict and bind, should be aware of something before they toss out *all* their bras : breast tissue, remember, is non-muscular, which also means it is non-elastic. The breasts are supported by tough inelastic tissue called Cooper's Ligaments. If your breasts are more than tiny, and you go without a bra, you may not boast a natural uplift for long. The continuous strain and pull of gravity on the breasts will stretch those ligaments and cause the breasts to sag. Once that happens, all the exercise in the world won't make the flesh firm again. You needn't wear a boned binder to keep you in shape, but you do need some gentle support. If your breasts are large and pendulous, a good supporting bra is absolutely essential except for those special occasions where a bounce is of the essence.

What is the point of including a chapter on breast exercises in this book? The point is that there are chest exercises you can do. The muscles underlying the breasts are your pectoral muscles; like any other they can be exercised to improve their tone and firm them up. Doing so *might* have some effect on the appearance of your breasts, but there is no guarantee.

Remember, too, that your pectoral muscles are your hugging muscles : any exercise you may do in that direction promises some happy fringe benefits !

1 HANDS CLASPED (good for starters)

Clasp your hands in front of you at chest level. Press them against each other as hard as you can. Hold for a count of five, then relax. Repeat five times. Progress by holding the contraction for a longer count as you feel your muscles increasing in strength. The more strength you gain, the harder you are able to resist yourself, and thus to build even more strength.

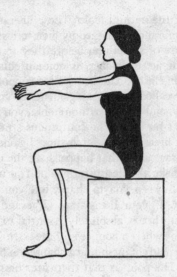

2 TWO HAND REACH (a variation)

Stretch both hands out in front of you at chest level, the backs of your hands touching. Press the backs of your hands together as hard as you can, and hold for the count of five. Repeat five times. Progress as above.

3 HANDS AT SIDE (another angle)

Drop both hands at your sides and place your hands against your thighs. With your hands and arms, press against your sides as hard as you can and tense your chest muscles. Hold for the count and relax. Repeat five times. Progress as above.

4 FOREARM CLUTCH (tricky but effective)

Clasp your hands in front of you about nose level, elbows bent and pointing down. Keep your forearms touching so that your elbows are together. Now press your forearms together as hard as possible. Hold for a count of five and relax. Repeat five times. Progress as above.

5 SCRUBBING FLOORS (it really works)

I hate to include this but it really happens to be great for the pectoral muscles – especially if the floors are really dirty. That may be some small consolation as you do the dirty deed.

For Men

A man's chest is unsightly and unattractive if it looks like it should be wearing a D cup. It's the rare woman who gets turned on by a man whose breast size rivals her own. Unlike a woman's, a man's chest should not have fatty and glandular development which makes for a feminine bustline. If you feel yourself bobbing as you run for the bus, you are probably overweight, with your pectoral, or chest, muscles in bad shape.

Masculine fat deposits tend to be on the chest and belly. Although exercise won't take the weight off, it *will* firm up the musculature underneath the fat and begin to make a more attractive appearance even before you lose some of those extra pounds through dieting.

A firm muscular chest is an asset on the beach and a definite plus in the bedroom. Achieving that desirable end is not a difficult feat. Here are some good chest exercises which can be performed without the use of equipment. They are the isometric type of exercise, which means that you provide your own resistance. The beauty of isometrics is that as your muscles develop and increase in strength, you are able to provide more resistance for yourself and thus to continue to increase in strength. You can also take your equipment with you, because all you really need is you!

1 HAND CLASP

Clasp your hands in front of you at chest level, elbows pointing out. As hard as you can, press your hands together and hold for a count of ten. Relax, then repeat ten times. Progress by increasing the count for the hold, then increasing the number of times you do the exercise.

2 WALL PRESS

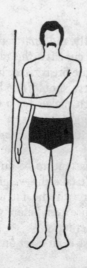

Stand with your left side against a wall. Crossing your right hand in front of you at chest level, place your palm against the wall at shoulder height. Press your hand against the wall as hard as you can and hold for a count of ten. Relax. Turn your right side to the wall and repeat with your left hand. Repeat. Progress as above.

3 FOREARM CLUTCH

Clasp your hands in front of you about nose level, elbows pointing down. Keep your forearms touching so that your elbows are together. Now press your forearms together as hard as possible. Hold for the count. Relax. Repeat. Progress as above.

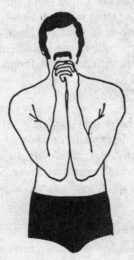

4 SIDE PRESS

Stand with your feet about eighteen inches apart. Bend forward from the waist, knees straight, and place your hands at the sides of your knees. Press your knees together as hard as you can with your hands and arms, and at the same time, resist the press with your knees. Hold the contraction for a count of ten. Relax and repeat. Progress as above.

If you have access to weights and pulleys, here's where you can put them to good use. You might find a stretch coil (chest expander) a good investment at this point if you're really serious.

5 USING WEIGHTS (If you haven't got weights, a heavy book will do)

Holding the weight in your right hand, put your arm at your side with your palm facing forward. Slowly lift your arm up and across your body until your nose touches your biceps. It is important to keep your elbow straight during this move. Lower slowly. Repeat with left hand. Progress as before.

6 USING A PULLEY

Begin by holding the pulley in your right hand with your arm lifted straight above you. Slowly pull down and across your body diagonally. Return slowly to starting position. Repeat with left hand. Progress as above. Start with fifteen times for each hand, and progress as you improve.

7 USING A STRETCH COIL (CHEST EXPANDER)

Tip: Begin by using only one coil and increasing to two, then three, when you feel your muscles are in good enough shape to be able to do the exercise very slowly. It is important that you, not the coils, are in control.

(a) Put the coil behind your back about level with your armpits. Keep your arms straight as you pull your arms together until your hands touch. Very slowly return to starting position.

(b) Hook one grip of your coil onto something stable such as the leg of a heavy bed. Lie down on your back and grip the other end. Keeping your elbow straight, pull the coil across your body. Slowly return to starting position. Repeat with other hand.

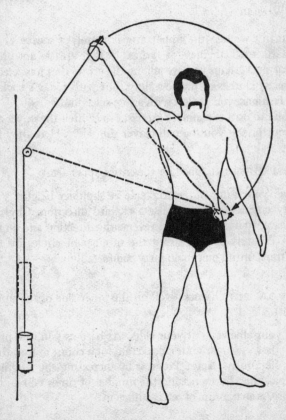

7 Arm Exercises

For Women

For many women the upper arm is merely a source of embarrassment. Flabbiness or fatness in that area is not pretty to look at. Perhaps you are among the group that has rejected sleeveless clothes as too revealing. But with today's backless bare fashions, you are left with a slim selection.

You can do a few simple exercises to tighten the upper arm without giving you football-player shoulders. Here they are.

1 ARM CIRCLING (good for the entire upper arm)

Stretch your arms out to the side at shoulder height. Very slowly circle your arms in a backward direction. Circle at least twenty-five times, then reverse the direction and go forward. Progress by increasing the number of circles by five each time, until you can do forty comfortably.

2 ELBOW PULL (works well on the inner side of the upper arm)

Tuck your elbows in at your sides. As hard as you can, press your elbows against your sides. Hold for a count of five, then relax. Repeat five times. Progress by increasing the length of the hold, then by increasing the number of times you do the exercise. A maximum of ten is sufficient.

3 BACKWARD PUSH (great for a flabby upper arm)

Stand with your back against a wall. Bend your arms at your sides so that your elbows touch the wall. Push your elbows backwards into the wall as hard as you can, and hold for a count of five. Progress as in 2.

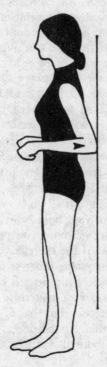

For Men

Fat may be the surplus of the Western world, but arms are not the usual place for an accumulation of fat in most men. Some men may have a flabby upper arm, but it is probably due to poor muscle tone in that area. Few men share the feminine concern that the bare look will ruin their social season !

In exercising your arms, you probably want to do more than just firm up flab, you want to build them up. If toning is enough for you, follow the exercises for women. Building muscle bulk is another story. To achieve an increase in bulk, you must work against a good amount of resistance as you exercise. You can do that by working against something immovable such as a wall, or by using weights or pulleys. This may be a good time to make a small investment in a stretch coil. Barbells are nice but not all that necessary when a small tote bag, packed with ever-increasing numbers of cans or amounts of sand, will do as well.

Here, then, is a group of exercises designed to build up the musculature of the arms and shoulders. Begin by doing those exercises you choose from each group five times, and hold each for a count of ten. If the exercise is performed against an immovable resistance, give it all your worth and progress by increasing the count of your hold by five each time, then by increasing the number of times you perform the exercise. The limit is up to you. If the exercise you have chosen uses weights or coils as resistance, progress by adding weight or coils, as well as increasing the length of your hold by five each time. You may also wish to increase the number of times you perform these exercises, but that depends on how much muscle you want to build. An increase to twenty-five times at most will probably be more than satisfactory.

Forearm Exercises

1 IMPOSSIBLE LIFT A

Sit at a desk or heavy table. Place your hands, palms up,

under the table and try to lift it. (If you can lift it, it's too light.) Hold for the count, then relax. Repeat.

2 IMPOSSIBLE LIFT B

Sitting as above, make fists of your hands and place them under the table, thumb side up. Try to lift the table with your fists. Progress as above.

3 IMPOSSIBLE LIFT C

Sitting as above, place the backs of your hands under the table and try to lift. Progress as above.

4 FOREARM RESIST

Sitting in a chair, place your left hand in your lap, palm side up. Put your right hand in your left. Try to bend your left hand at the wrist and elbow, but use your right hand to prevent any movement. Hold for the count, then relax and reverse hands. Repeat. Progress as above.

5 FOREARM RESIST VARIATION

Sitting in a chair as above, place your left hand in your lap, palm side down. Place your right hand on top. Attempt to extend your left wrist, but prevent any movement of your left hand with pressure from your right. Hold and count, then relax. Reverse hands and repeat.

Upper Arm Exercises

1 ELBOW RESIST

Sitting in a chair, place your left hand on your lap, palm up. Put your right hand on your left arm just below the elbow.

Attempt to bend your left elbow, but prevent any movement with pressure from your right hand. Hold and count. Relax. Reverse hands and repeat.

2 LEG LIFT

Sitting in a chair, place both hands under your thighs. Try to lift your legs. Hold and count, then relax. Repeat.

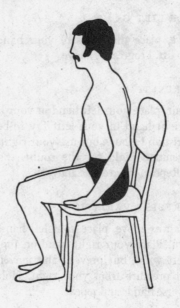

3 ELBOW EXTENSION

Sitting at a desk or table, place both hands on the table in front of you, palm sides up. Press firmly into the table as though to straighten your arms, but the table will prevent any movement. Hold and count. Relax. Repeat.

4 TWO ARM DOUBLECROSS

Cross your arms in front of you at the wrists. Turn the palms together towards each other so that you can clasp them together. Press your palms together so that your right hand is pulling towards the right, your left hand to the left. Hold for the count, then relax. Repeat.

5 BICEPS BUILDER (using weights)

Holding a weight in your right hand, keep your arm close to your side and lift the weight by bending your elbow. Lift slowly, then lower slowly. Repeat with the same arm until you have completed the required number of lifts. Now change hands and repeat exercise. Progress as indicated in the text.

6 BICEPS PULL (using coils)

Stand up and put one grip of the coil spring under your right foot. Hold the other grip in your right hand, palm facing upward, and bend your hand towards your shoulder. Release the coil very slowly. Repeat with the right hand until you have completed the required number of pulls. Then do the exercise with your left arm. Progress as indicated in the text.

Shoulder Exercises

1 SIT LIFT

Sitting in a chair, place both hands on either side of the chair and grip the seat. Try to lift your seat off the chair. Hold for the count, then relax. Repeat.

2 WALL PUSH

Stand very close to a wall, facing it, and put both hands on the wall. Attempt to push yourself away from the wall, using your arms, but use your body to prevent any movement. Press as hard as you can, hold, then relax. Repeat. Progress.

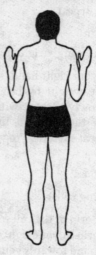

3 PUSH-UPS

Lying face down on the floor, try to do your push-ups from your toes. If you are unable to push off with your toes, use your knees, but when that becomes easy, progress to toes. Begin with five push-ups and increase the number to progress *ad infinitum.*

4 DOORWAY REACH

Stand in a doorway and touch the sides with the backs of your hands. Pressing as hard as you can, attempt to widen the doorway. Hold for the count, then relax. Repeat.

5 BACKWARD WALL PRESS

Stand with your back to a wall. Put your elbows against the wall, and attempt to push yourself away from the wall by pressing with your elbows. Use your body weight to prevent any movement. Hold and count. Relax. Repeat.

6 CHIN-UPS

Note: This is a very strenuous exercise, and should be attempted only when you know you are in good shape. It requires strong shoulders and a good heart.
Using a bar or door frame above you, grip the bar with your palms facing towards you. Lift your entire body until your chin reaches the bar. Progress by increasing the number of times you perform the exercise.

7 STRAIGHT ARM LIFT A (using weights)

Holding the weight in your right hand, keep your elbow straight, and raise your arm in front of you all the way up. Lower slowly. Repeat the exercise the required number of times with your right arm, then transfer the weight and perform the exercise with your left arm. Repeat the exercise ten times with each arm, and progress as the exercise becomes easier.

8 STRAIGHT ARM LIFT B (using weights)

Standing as above, raise your right arm and weight out to the side, remembering to keep your elbow straight. When you reach shoulder level, turn your palm up and continue raising your arm above your head. To lower, reverse the procedure. Repeat the required number of times, then transfer the weight and do the exercise with your left arm. Progress as above.

9 STRAIGHT ARM LIFT C (using weights)

Standing as above, and keeping your elbow straight, lift your right arm behind you. Repeat the required number of times, then transfer the weight and repeat with your left arm. Progress as indicated.

10 STRAIGHT ARM CIRCLING (using weights)

Holding the weight in your right hand, take your arm out to the side with a straight elbow, and make slow circles. Begin by doing ten circles with your right hand, then transfer the weight and repeat with your left arm. Progress by increasing the number of circles by five each time. You may also increase the weight.

11 COIL STRETCH (using a coil spring)

Stand up and hold the coil in front of you. With straight elbows, stretch the coil apart until your arms are at your sides at shoulder level. It is important to return to the starting position very slowly (don't let the coil snap back). If you can't release it slowly, wait until your shoulders are stronger.

12 BACK COIL STRETCH (using a coil spring)

Put the coil spring behind your back. Hold the grips one in each hand, and keep your elbows straight. Move your arms forward until your hands touch in front. Release *very* slowly.

13 DELTOID PULL (using a coil spring)

Stand on one grip of the coil with your right foot. Hold the other grip with your right hand. Keep your elbow straight and stretch the coil out as far as possible to the side. Release slowly. Repeat the required number of times, then transfer to the other side and repeat again. Progress as indicated.

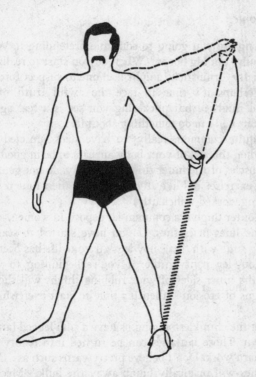

Tip: Swimming is a great shoulder builder. The resistance of the water, especially when working for speed, helps develop good muscle.

8 Thigh Exercises

For Women

How long are you going to continue pretending to yourself that you've got big bones? When do you start to realize that those hefty 'drumsticks' might lead one to suspect force feeding? Perhaps it's time to face the awful truth of slack muscled thighs: that puckering you see is a real age giveaway. But you *can* do something about it.

It's quite common, really, to have slack muscled thighs even when the rest of your body appears to be in good shape. The muscles of the inner thigh, especially, do not get a great deal of exercise, and like any others, lose their tone if they're not being worked sufficiently.

The outer thigh is a common fat deposit in women, and can ruin the lines of clothes. If you have started to search for bathing suits with 'little-boy legs'; if your life has been saved by a long-leg panty-girdle; if you're beginning to wonder when the inner sides of your rubbing thighs will show telltale signs of erosion – then it's time to start exercising your thighs.

Even the chunkiest among us have a slim-legged fantasy of our own. Those fantasies can be turned into reality with a little hard work. Don't believe pretty yarns such as: 'Mighty machines will magically bump away the bulk.' 'Mechanical shaker-uppers invisibly slim you down.' It just isn't so. You have to work your own muscles to tone them up. It takes a little effort to achieve results, but the results will be real, and you'll be able to see the difference yourself, not just on a chart but in the mirror where it counts — your own secret dream come true.

Before you panic and begin to wonder just how much work there *really* is, look through the following exercises. They are all quite easy and effective. Choose the ones you like best and go to it.

1 LEG SWING (very good for the outer thigh)

Lie on the floor on your side. Bend your bottom hip and knee for balance. Lift your top leg up about eighteen inches. Move your top leg slowly forwards, then backwards, then back to the centre and down. Repeat ten times. Change sides and exercise the other leg. Progress by increasing the number of times you exercise each leg.

2 LEG CIRCLING (a variation of 1 with the same effect)

Lie on the floor as above. Raise your upper leg and make large slow circles going clockwise ten times. Without resting the leg, reverse the circle for another ten times. Change sides and repeat with the other leg. Progress by increasing the number of circles for each leg.

3 BATHTIME SLIMMER (do this in the bath – relaxing and slimming all in one)

Sitting in the bath, spread your legs so they touch the sides of the bath. Press your legs into the sides of the bath (keeping your knees straight) as hard as you can, and hold for a count of ten. Relax. Repeat the exercise ten times. Progress by increasing the length of the hold until you can reach twenty-five, then increase the number of times you do the exercise.

4 WALL PRESS (an outer thigh firmer-upper)

Stand about a foot away from a wall with your side to the wall. Hold onto the wall to steady yourself. Raise the leg nearest the wall sideways so that you press against the wall as hard as you can. Hold for a count of ten. Relax. Repeat ten times. Then change sides and repeat the exercise with the other leg. Progress by increasing the length of the hold, then by increasing the number of times you do the exercise.

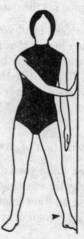

5 TAILOR SITTING PRESS (great for outer thighs and buttocks)

Sit on the floor in crossed leg position. Hold your hands under your knees. With your hands try to pull your knees together, but at the same time press down with your knees to prevent any movement. Press down as hard as you can, and hold for a count of ten. Do the exercise ten times if you can. Progress by increasing the length of the hold, then increasing the number of times you perform the exercise.

6 TAILOR SITTING PUSH-UPS (a winner for the inner thigh)

Sit in crossed leg position on the floor. Put your hands on top of your knees. With your legs try to pull your knees together, but use your hands as resistance to prevent any movement. Push up with your knees as hard as possible, and hold for a count of ten. Repeat ten times. Progress as in 5.

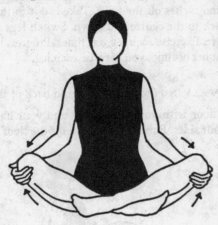

7 BOOK PRESS (easy and effective, for the inner thigh)

Lie on your back with your knees bent and your feet flat on the floor. Place a book between your knees (the thicker the better). Press your knees together into the book as hard as you can, and hold for ten. Relax. Repeat ten times. Progress as above.

8 KNEE CLINCHER (to tighten a slack inner thigh)

Sit on the floor with your knees bent and your feet flat on the floor. Hold your knees together, but use your hands (or some-

one else's) to try to pry them apart. Hold for the count. Relax.
Repeat. Progress as above.

9 STRAIGHT LEG RAISE (to shape up the front of your
thighs)

Lie on your back and bend your left knee so the foot is flat on
the floor. Keep your right knee straight and lift your right
leg about ten inches off the floor. Take it out to the right, to
the left, back to the centre and down. Switch legs and repeat
with the left. Exercise each leg ten times. Progress by increasing the number of times you exercise each leg.

10 CRAB WALKING (good for front and back of the thigh)

Sit on the floor with your knees bent and your hands palms
down at your sides. Raise your bottom off the floor as high as

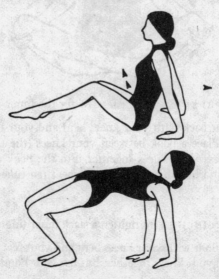

you can, so that you are on your hands and feet. Now walk backwards. Begin by walking for about thirty seconds, and increase the time until you can walk about three minutes.

11 DEEP KNEE BEND (an oldy but goody, for the front of the thigh)

Do this beside a table so that you have support if you need it. First up on your toes, then slowly bend your knees until you reach a squatting position. Slowly back to standing. Repeat five times, and increase as you are able.

12 KNEE SITTING (a great thigh exercise, a tummy tightener too)

Get down on your knees and sit on your heels. Reach both hands out in front of you, and lift your seat off your heels. Now keep your trunk straight, and lean backwards at a forty-five degree angle. Hold for a count of ten if possible. Relax.

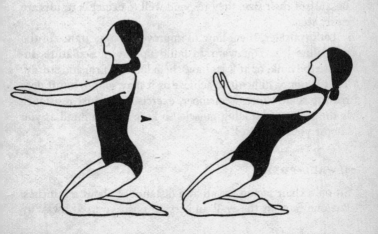

Repeat if you can. Progress by increasing the length of the count, then by increasing the number of times you do the exercise, as tolerated.

For Men

A common site for fatty deposits in the female is the thigh, but that just isn't so for most men. More likely you are dissatisfied with your legs because they are too thin for the rest of you. They're not developed enough, it seems, not enough bulk, and you may even wonder how they manage to get you around without buckling under the strain. If you're thin, then lanky limbs are almost acceptable. But there's nothing more comical than the chubby man whose watermelon waistline is balanced atop a pair of toothpick legs.

The muscles along the front aspect of the thigh are called the quadriceps, and they are really massive. They're large, long, built for heavy work. Just walking around from here to there is not enough to keep them in tip-top condition. Because of their size, they respond well to exercise; results are easily seen.

Let's consider, then, how to improve the appearance of the masculine leg. You want to build up the musculature, increase the bulk, or at least have them looking firm and sturdy. That is not as difficult to achieve as it may sound, but it does require some effort. Remember, exercising against resistance is the secret of building muscle, so keep that in mind as you choose your exercises.

1 WALL PUSH

Sit on a chair facing a wall at a distance of about ten inches. Put one foot on the wall and try to push yourself away by attempting to straighten your knee. Don't allow any movement. Push for a count of ten. Relax and repeat with the other leg. Repeat the exercise ten times for each leg. Progress by increasing the hold of the contraction and increasing the number of times you perform the exercise.

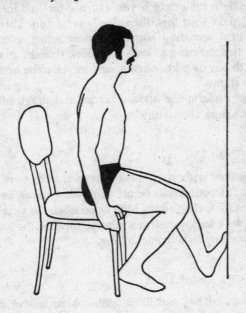

2 STEPPING UP

Using a sturdy chair or suitably high box, step onto it and down ten times, leading with your right foot. Then repeat, leading with your left foot. Begin by doing the exercise ten times with each leg, and progress by increasing the number of times.

Climbing stairs three at a time has somewhat the same effect.

Note: This is a strenuous exercise, so if you have a weak heart, omit it.

3 DEEP KNEE BEND

Stand beside a table which you can use for balance if you need it. Up on your toes, then slowly bend your knees until you are in a squatting position. Slowly return to starting position, remembering to keep your back straight as you do. Begin with ten deep knee bends, and increase the number as tolerance allows.

Variation: Perform the above exercise and progressions on one leg at a time, alternating legs.

4 CRAB WALKING

Sit on the floor with your knees bent so your feet are flat on the floor. Put your hands beside you, palms down, and raise your bottom off the floor as high as possible. On your hands and feet, walk backwards for a minute. Increase the length of time for walking, as tolerance allows.

5 STRAIGHT LEG RAISE

Take a handled bag and fill it with ten pounds of cans or sand. Lie on your back, with your left knee bent so that the foot is flat on the floor. Hook the handle of the weighted bag over your right ankle. Keep your right knee straight, and lift the leg about ten inches. Hold for a count of ten and lower slowly. Repeat with the same leg ten times. Then transfer the bag and exercise the left leg the same way. Progress by increasing the length of the hold, by increasing the number of times you do the exercise, and then by adding to the weights in the bag.

6 COSSACK STEP

Squat in a doorway with your hands holding the frame for balance. Straighten one knee so your heel is on the floor. Now hop to change legs and continue doing so fifteen times. Progress by increasing the number of leg changes.

7 DUCK WALKING

Squat down, put your hands on your hips, and walk. Begin by walking for two minutes. Progress by increasing the length of your walk as tolerated.

8 BIKE RIDING

This needs no explanation, but it's handy to know that the more resistance you have, the harder your legs must work, and that is good for muscle building.

9 KNEE SITTING

Get down on your knees and sit on your heels. Reach both hands out in front of you, and lift your seat off your heels.

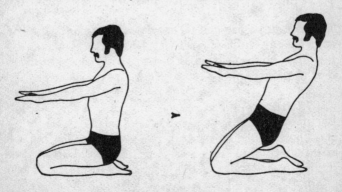

Keep your trunk straight, and lean back at a forty-five degree angle. Hold for a count of ten. Return to starting position. Repeat five times. Progress by increasing the length of the hold by five each time, and by increasing the number of times you perform the exercise.

You can make this exercise more difficult by keeping your hands on your hips as you lean back.

9 Buttock Exercises

There's nothing quite so unappealing as a woman who's too broad in the beam. Are *you* one of those delightful ladies who furtively hide behind dressing room curtains, and in the darkness switch the bottom half of a pants suit so discreetly that only you know you have matched a size eighteen lower to go with the size twelve upper?

Or are you a man whose cherubic cheeks look like the devil from the rear? A shiny seat is a sinful necessity of life if you're a gentleman who jellos as he jogs.

If any of these unhappy descriptions has a familiar ring, then it's time to take action. If you're somewhat overweight, and nature has chosen your buttocks as a convenient spot to store the extra fat, don't despair: underneath is a pair of massive muscles, and just tightening them up may actually take inches off your measurements.

These muscles, the gluteus maximus, respond well to exercise as they are large and built for work. Don't fool yourself into believing that the running you do all day, downstairs to the laundry and upstairs to search for the orphaned sock, is enough to keep you in shape. It's not. But following a simple routine of buttock exercises may get you back on the whistle list.

If you do have some weight to lose, a combination of diet *and* exercise can do wonderful things. Remember, dieting alone is not selective, but if you exercise too, you have some control over the outcome.

If you're simply flabby, you needn't diet. Exercise alone will achieve the end you had in mind.

Here then are some good exercises for the buttocks.

1 SINGLE LEG LIFT (a good tightener)

Lie on the floor face down and hands under your forehead. With your knees straight, lift your right leg, *keeping* your knee straight. Hold for a count of five and lower slowly. Repeat with your left leg. Exercise each leg five times to begin. Progress by increasing the length of the hold until you can hold for a count of twenty, and then by increasing the number of times you perform the exercise.

2 DOUBLE LEG LIFT (a progression of 1 and *very* strenuous; not to be done by anyone with a bad back)

Lie on the floor as above. Lift both legs keeping the knees straight, and hold for the count. Progress as above.

3 THE RAINBOW (tough but worth the effort)

Lie on your back with your elbows bent at a right angle. Tighten your hips and back muscles. Slowly arch your back by pushing off at elbows, head, and heels. Hold and count. Relax. Begin by doing the exercise three times. Progress as above.

4 CRAB WALKING (cute and effective)

Sit on the floor and bend your knees so that your feet are flat on the floor. Put your hands beside you, palms down on the floor. Now raise your bottom off the floor so that you are on your hands and feet. Walk forward, keeping your middle section as high as possible. Count about twenty-five steps, and then walk backwards. Progress by increasing the number of steps you take.

5 WALL PRESS (easy and it works)

Stand with your back to a wall. Press your right leg into the wall as hard as you can, remembering to keep your leg straight. Hold and count as you tighten your buttocks. Relax and repeat with the other leg. Begin by working each leg five

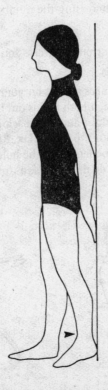

times and holding for a count of five. Progress by increasing the length of the hold, then increasing the number of times you perform the exercise.

6 SEAT WALKING (anyone can do it)

Sit on the floor with your legs straight out in front of you. Lifting one hip slightly off the floor, move that leg forward, then alternate so that you are walking on your seat. Walk about twenty-five steps in this manner, and then walk backwards. Progress by increasing the number of steps you take.

7 KNEE SITTING (strong exercise for entire upper thighs and buttocks)

Get down on your knees and sit on your heels. Lift your seat off your heels and reach both hands out in front of you. Now, keep your trunk straight and lean back at a forty-five degree angle. Hold it and count to ten. Relax. Repeat if you can. Progress by increasing the length of the hold, and increasing the number of times you do the exercise as tolerated.

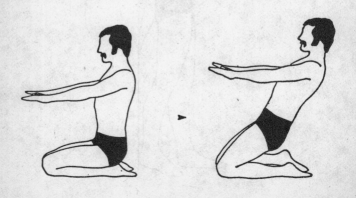

10 Exercises for the Back of the Legs

Right behind your knees is a group of muscles called the hamstrings. Their main job is to bend your knees, but they also contribute to the soft curve at the back above your knees. In some parts of the world it's considered terribly *risqué* to show the hollow behind the knees which is defined by the hamstrings. In our part of the world, however, a girl who *doesn't* expose this little bit of anatomy may be suspected of having something awful to hide.

How are your hamstrings? Worthy of a whistle? Do they entice an enviable following? If not, perhaps you'd like to try a few exercises to tone them up. Here are a few you can do to gentle that curve and highlight that hollow.

1 CRAB WALKING (firms up the whole rear view)

Sit on the floor with your knees bent and your feet flat on the floor. Place your hands beside you, palms down. Now raise your bottom up off the floor, as high as you can, so that you are on your hands and feet, and walk forwards. Keep walking for one minute. Progress by increasing your time of walking, as tolerated.

2 BOTTOM CREEPING (good for the hamstrings and stomach too)

Sit on the floor with your legs straight out in front of you.

Now dig in with your heels and pull your body towards your feet, bending your knees and sliding your bottom along the floor as you do so. Repeat the exercise ten times. Progress by increasing the number of times you do the exercise.

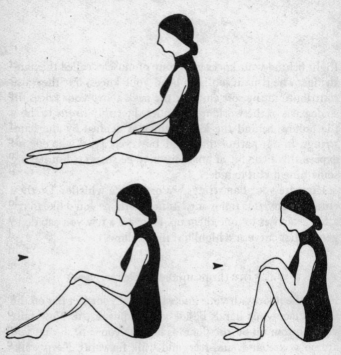

3 FLUTTER KICK (a bottom bonus in this one)

Lie on your stomach and rest your head on your hands. Alternating your legs, kick your feet to your seat without letting them touch the floor. Begin by exercising for one minute, and progress by increasing the length of time you continue the kicking.

11 Waistline Exercises

Your weight isn't really too bad; your bottom half isn't yet included on the nation's list of disaster areas; your upper section even rates an occasional whistle. But somewhere in the middle it all goes to pot.

Perhaps you see red when the alterations lady suggests that you keep the dress but consider easing it out around the middle; or when your sweetheart tells you that it's great to have something to grab onto, not like those wispy little creatures with no waist at all.

Don't panic. There's hardly a woman around who can't do with a little waist whittling. A thickening waist is a problem common in menopausal women, but by no means restricted to them. It's basically due to poor muscle tone, a condition shared by young women too. Poor muscle tone is correctable through proper exercise. All you need do is do it.

If you are a bona fide member of the middle-muddle sisterhood, no matter what your age or stage, the first thing to do is stop blaming your mother. True, heredity does have some influence on your shape, but it's *not* her fault that you have gone and lost it. Whatever your bone structure, there is always some room for improvement, and here's your opportunity to stop paying dues where you receive no dividends.

Have a good look at yourself in the mirror. If your middle is really a mess, you had better start off with some abdominal exercises to tighten you up. You will find them in Chapter Three. Choose a few good ones and get to work: they will pay off. Combine them with the following exercises designed to whittle your waist. Then you have a programme that is going to work on your problem area.

If your stomach is flat and your abdominals strong, and it's just a matter of aiming for a narrow waist, omit the abdominal exercises and just do the waist whittlers. They're easy, they're safe, and they work. Begin by doing each five times, unless otherwise indicated, and hold for a count of five. Progress by increasing the length of the hold, and then by increasing the number of times you perform the exercise.

1 CROSS KNEE REACH (good for starters)

Lie on the floor on your back, and bend your knees so that your feet are flat on the floor. With your right hand reach to the outside of your left knee, and lift your head and shoulders up off the floor. Hold for the count and lower slowly. Repeat with your left hand reaching to the outside of your right knee. Repeat five times.

2 ELBOW REACH (a progression of 1, harder, but better if you are really up to it)

Lying on the floor as above, place your hands behind your head. Reach with your right elbow towards your left knee. Hold for the count, then lower slowly. Repeat with your left elbow to your right knee. Repeat five times.

3 SIDE STRETCHER (a real waistline wonder)

Lie on your back with your hands at your sides. Lift your head and shoulders just slightly off the floor. With your right hand, reach sideways towards your right knee. Slowly return to the centre, and without resting, reach your left hand towards your left knee. Back to the centre, then rest. Repeat five times.

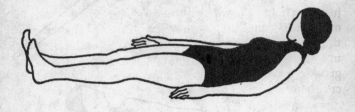

4 HIP RAISING

Lie on your back with your hands at your sides. Raise your right hip as though trying to shorten your leg. Return to starting position and repeat with your left leg. Repeat at least ten times for each leg. Progress to twenty-five times.

5 SIDE LYING STRETCH (not for back ache sufferers)

Lie on your left side with your left hand out for balance. Keep your legs straight and in line with your torso. Reach your right hand down towards your right knee. Hold for the count. Return to starting position and rest. Repeat five times, then change sides and repeat exercise, stretching with your left hand. (See diagram p. 94.)

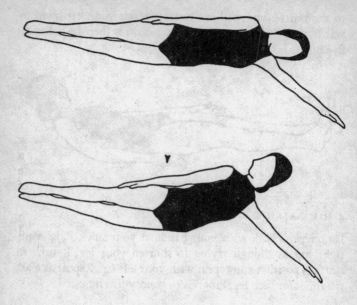

How you treat your feet may have a direct bearing on how the rest of you feels. If everything but your feet feels like a million, there's an appreciable decrease in your spendable energy. It's hard to hobble your way through the time of your life.

How you choose to dress your feet has a great deal to do with how your feet treat you. If I didn't know better, I would suspect the shoe manufacturers of being in league with orthopaedists, chiropodists, and all the other foot fixers, whose offices are lately stuffed with shoe freaks. A lot of today's fashionable footwear seems created solely to cramp your style. Knowing what happens to your feet when they are poorly shod may save you time and tears, and allow your feet to become a form of transportation you had long forgotten.

A normal foot is composed of twenty-six bones, their associated joints, and many muscles and ligaments which tie it up in a neat little package. Unless you have a structural abnormality, your foot has two arches, one longitudinal and one transverse. These arches are maintained by the muscles and tendons around the foot, by the form of the bones themselves, and by ligaments and other tissue. The whole design has three main functions:

(1) It helps to distribute your body weight evenly, so that no part of the foot is under excess strain.

(2) It gives spring and elasticity to your step.

(3) It helps to break the shock when you are running or jumping.

The reason I've bothered to include all this technical matter is to make it clear that the common foot is truly an outstanding engineering design. The whole thing is beautifully balanced to provide maximum effectiveness with a minimum of effort. And it is this careful balance we so callously disregard when selecting our shoes.

Let me begin by emphatically stating that 'barefoot is healthy'. Without the confines of a shoe, your foot is able to adjust to the surface on which you are standing, distribute your weight properly, and give you all the traction you require. If it wasn't that our paths are strewn with potentially dangerous prickles (and a little snow now and again), there would be no need for shoes at all. Many barefoot natives have stronger, healthier and happier feet than we do – feet that are capable of fantastic feats – all for the want of shoes.

How, then, do we choose a shoe that is safe, sensible, but doesn't look like the old school oxford? A few basic facts should make it all clear.

When your heel is raised more than one and a half or two inches above the forefoot, your body weight is thrust forward, putting tremendous pressure on the forefoot and disturbing the balance of weight distribution. The result can be sore feet or worse. Continuous pressure of this kind can lead to bunions, calluses, and generally unattractive feet so common in middle-aged women. With the unsightliness comes pain. A sensible height of heel is, then, an important consideration in choosing a shoe that you plan to wear a lot. If once in a while you want to kick up your four-inch heels, you probably won't suffer for it, but it doesn't make sense for everyday wear.

Your feet, you may have noticed, have a special talent. They react to excess pressure or rubbing by forming a thickening of the skin, or callus, for self-protection. Sounds good.

But a really tough callus can be painful too, like walking around with a pebble in your shoe. The fit of your shoe is important, then. You want to find one with some good wiggling room for your toes, but which will still grip your heel firmly without rubbing. It's a real art.

When your shoes, stretch socks, or stockings are too short, you're asking for crooked toes. The tendons of your toes, no longer having room to stretch, will shorten out of laziness.

For safety's sake, choose a shoe with some traction if it is to be worn most often on carpeted areas, especially around the house. It's also good practice to leave your mules at the top of the stairs, or you may find you have 'slipped into' something you hadn't counted on.

Sandals are great if they don't cut or bind. Clogs are fine too as long as you *don't* wear them with stockings.

Footwear faddists, beware the four-inch heel. In order for you to balance on them, it's almost mandatory to throw your back out of alignment. As well, your toes are thrust forward with an incredible amount of stress.

Platforms are another story. Most of them don't have the heel raised too high in relation to the forefoot, so you're safe on that score. But are you *really* safe venturing out into the big wide world on them? Unless you are especially nimble-footed, and can do a good balancing act, you had better forgo their dubious pleasures; the prospect of an occasional turned ankle may be imminent. Not all platforms are that unwieldy: some are attractive and quite easy to manoeuvre. Just use your head and save your feet.

Choosing your shoes intelligently is one good way to look after your feet. Exercising them is another.

You bother to exercise your feet because all the usual running of the day is not enough. Exercise improves their condition so that you tire less easily. If you have a job that demands you stand rooted to the spot like a potted plant, you exercise to increase the circulation in your feet, and thus their stamina. You also bother to exercise to strengthen your foot muscles and so maintain the balance which makes for proper weight distribution. Keeping your feet in healthy condition makes you feel better generally.

You're probably wondering about exercising as a method to improve the shape of your calf and ankle. Unless you're grossly overweight, your ankles are defined by the bony structure and tendon attachments beneath the skin, and there is not much you can do about that. If you have heavy calves, exercise will tighten and tone them, but it's not likely to decrease their bulk. If your calves are too thin, however, you can build up your calf muscles through exercise, and work your way to a more pleasing contour. As you move towards more shapely calves, you improve the appearance of your ankles as well.

Here, then, is a list of exercises for your lower leg. Choose the ones you like best .

1 ANKLE CIRCLING (great for calves and feet; the pumping action of the calf muscles helps improve the circulation in the whole leg)

Sitting on a chair, straighten your right leg out in front of you. Turning from the ankle, make small circles with your foot. Go clockwise twenty-five times, then reverse direction for twenty-five more turns. Repeat with the left foot. Progress to fifty circles each way.

2 BIG TOE SIDE STEP (It's tough to get the hang of this one, but it is good for the small muscles of the forefoot, especially if you have a tendency to bunions.)

Sitting on a chair, put both feet on the floor about four inches apart and parallel. Moving the big toes only, try to move each big toe towards the other. When you have moved them, hold for a count of five, then relax. Repeat five times. Progress to holding for a count of ten, then increasing the number of times you perform the exercise.

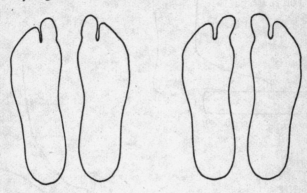

3 TOWEL SHUFFLE (good for the small muscles of the foot, strengthening them and restoring muscle balance)

Put a towel on the floor and sit on a chair. Using your right foot, gather the towel up in your toes, but try not to curl your toes. Rather, keep your toes straight, and bend at the joint comparable to the knuckle joint of the hand. When you have gone the length of the towel, repeat with the left foot. Progress by increasing the number of times you perform the exercise.

4 BOOK LIFT (good for the whole lower leg, as it works on the calves and Achilles tendon)

Put a book about two inches thick on the floor. Stand on it with the front half of your foot only, letting your heels hang over the edge. Now, up on your toes. Lower yourself slowly until your heels are touching the floor. Return slowly to starting position. Repeat five times. Progress by increasing the number of times you perform the exercise.

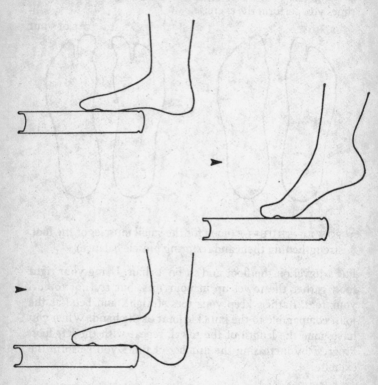

5 WALKING (just the way it sounds – a top-notch exercise for legs, feet, ankles, and all the rest of you)

The secret of walking to gain real benefits is not to saunter or meander. Taking your time, or just going for a stroll, is more tiring than not. To use walking as an exercise for your legs and heart, you want to walk at an even pace, quick but comfortable. You want to 'hit your stride'. It really does wonders for generally improving your feeling of well being. Even if you are going to walk only a short distance, make it worthwhile, make it brisk. But if you can, make it a part of your daily routine, and put your heart into it.

13 Limbering-up Exercises

Most exercise books you'll find on the market, most television programmes for exercising ladies, seem to be obsessed with muscle-stretching exercises. They call it limbering up. But muscle-stretching is what it is.

Most of us grew up under the misconception that stretching our muscles does wonderful things. It really doesn't, it only stretches them. Somewhere we believed that to be 'double-jointed' was to be lucky. To be able to sling your leg around your neck was to be admired. To be able to slide your head between your legs, backwards, was a gift. To touch your thumb to your forearm was a talent.

If you are an ordinary human being, concerned with being in good physical condition and looking your best, there is really no need to be an amateur acrobat. If you're an athlete, or really have an interest in pursuing an active sport, it's quite another story.

An athlete or a participant in active games needs to be loose – not as an added measure to his skill or stamina, but as a form of self-protection. Being limber can make the difference between injury or safety in a fall or an uncontrolled movement. It gives you extra leeway, so to speak, before you tear a muscle or ligament, by making a larger range of movement available to you. A skier, a tennis player, a skater, or any participant in a sport where pulled muscles are the order of the day, would do himself a favour to limber up, or stretch his muscles.

In this chapter I have selected a group of exercises specifically designed with the active sportsman in mind. These exercises will not build muscle power, strength, or endurance, but they will put a stretch on those muscles most likely to be tight, and therefore easily injured when suddenly pulled in a slip, a fall, or any unanticipated movement. They are safe in that you won't hurt your back when you perform them, but you will probably feel stiff for the first few days. If you do, try to work through the stiffness until you can perform the exercise comfortably. Remember that hot baths are relaxing to tired muscles.

Do all the exercises slowly, avoiding quick jerky movements, and feel a good pull on the muscles involved. Progress by attempting to increase your range of movement each time you try.

1 CALF STRETCH #1

Place a book about two inches thick on the floor. Stand on it with the front half of your feet, letting your heels hang over the edge. Slowly rise up on your toes, then slowly lower yourself until your heels touch the floor. Return to starting position. Repeat ten times.

2 CALF STRETCH #2

Standing upright, place your right foot well behind you and lower your heel to the floor. Bend your left knee and, putting your hands on it for support, lean forward. Remember to keep your right heel touching the ground. Hold for a count of five, then return to standing. Repeat the exercise reversing the

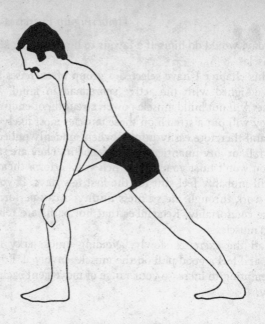

position of your legs so that your left foot is behind you. Exercise each leg five times.

3 HAMSTRING STRETCH #1

Sit on the floor with both legs straight in front of you. Using your hands to grasp your legs below the knees, crawl forward with your hands trying to reach your feet. When you can do that comfortably, progress by trying to get your head down to touch your knees.

4 HAMSTRING STRETCH #2

Sit on the floor with your legs spread apart. Reach your right hand down to grasp your ankle, and try to get your right ear to touch that knee. Hold the position, then return to sitting, and repeat for the left side. Work each side five times, each time getting your ear closer to your knee.

5 HAMSTRING STRETCH #3

Stand up straight with your feet about eighteen inches apart. Raise both hands above your head, and arch your back so that

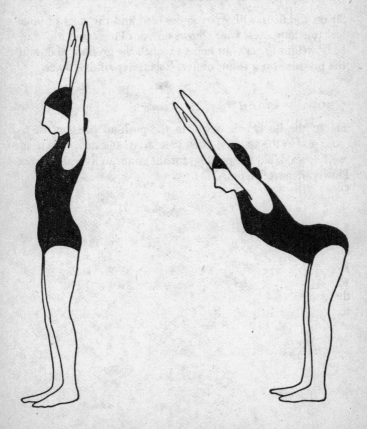

you stick your bottom out. Now slowly lean forward, keeping your back arched and your hands raised. You will feel the pull almost immediately, so take it easy and don't overdo. Your final aim is to have your body at right angles to your legs, but that will take time. Repeat the exercise five times and rest.

6 INNER THIGH STRETCH

Sit on the floor with your knees bent and the soles of your feet touching. Rest your elbows on your knees, and use your body weight to get your knees to touch the ground. Maintain the pressure for a count of five. Relax. Repeat five times.

7 BODY STRETCH

Lie on the floor, face down, in the push-up position. Raise your seat in the air, straighten your arms, and tuck your head well down. Hold the position for the count of five, and lower slowly. Repeat five times.

14 Bedroom Bonus

Liberating your libido may actually be the next-best thing to a few laps around the track! It's really quite true. For starters, regular love-making is an A-1 exercise for your heart and lungs. Sexual activity increases pulse and respiration, and when, like any exercise programme, it is followed with some regularity, it strengthens the heart muscle, improves circulation, and improves lung capacity.

You'll be happy to know, too, that making love is a terrific body toner. You are actively involving all your major muscle groups in strenuous exercise; if done often enough, you'll actually benefit by improving your shape.

If you're beneath your partner, make it work for you. All that pelvic thrusting against a resistant weight does wonders for your buttocks and abdominal muscles. Using your legs for squeezing, aside from the obvious pleasure, is terrific exercise for the upper thighs. Your upper arms and chest get a good work-out when you make your hugging felt, even the little muscles of your back are brought into play if you get right into the act.

When on top of your partner, you accrue the same interest with perhaps a little extra bonus for your thighs.

The variations in position are endless, and so are the benefits.

15 Exercising in the Water

Water has long been thought of as a universal panacea, better even than an aspirin. If your feet ache, you soak them. A long hot bath performs minor miracles for your aching back or tired limbs. Today the whirlpool bath adds yet another valuable medium available to therapists and doctors for treatment of limbs and body. In the therapeutic pool, many a weakened or paralysed muscle has made its first move towards recovery.

As a way to play, or a means to a medal, water offers a myriad of experiences, and is used by everyone from infants to the aged. It's fun, it's refreshing, it's exhausting and exhilarating. It's also an outstanding exercise medium.

Using the buoyancy of water, one can perform fantastic feats. Muscles can relax and use minimal effort to achieve movement. But – and here's the clincher – water can be used effectively as a resistance. That it why very good swimmers are in such fantastic shape. They are working their muscles against the resistance of the water; as a result, they improve in tone, strength, and endurance. The more you increase the speed of the movement you are performing in water, the greater the effective resistance encountered.

Swimming at a good pace is a great way to get your body into shape. Shoulders, legs and buttocks particularly are built up with the conventional kind of water work. But if you know how to position yourself in the water, you can exercise any muscle group you choose. As your muscles begin to shape up, you will be able to increase the speed of the exercise, and thus increase the resistance against which you are working.

Here are some good pool exercises designed for specific muscle groups. Choose the ones best suited to your own trouble spots and do each one five times, as quickly as you can. You will progress by increasing the speed of your movement as your strength improves, and by increasing the number of times you perform the exercise. For some, increasing the depth of the water in which you are working adds resistance, and you will find that indicated in the exercise.

1 RUNNING IN WATER (great exercise for the entire leg)

In shallow water, run as quickly as you can from one side of the pool to the other. Try to get your knees up as high as possible. Progress by increasing your speed and by increasing the depth of the water in which you are running. Running in deep water also provides good work for your abdominal muscles.

2 SPREAD EAGLE (terrific for the entire upper leg and thigh)

Stand facing the side of the pool in water up to your chest. Get a good grip on the side of the pool for support, and keep your back straight. As quickly as you can, spread your legs wide. Now, very quickly, snap them back together. You will feel your muscles working hard against the water. Repeat five times. Progress as tolerated.

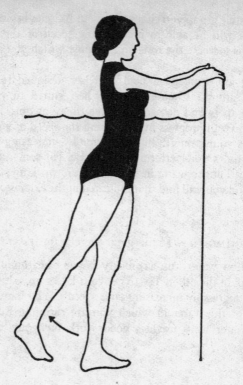

3 BACK KICK (a good buttock tightener, and stomach toner too)

Facing the side of the pool and standing close to it in chest-high water, grip the pool side firmly. As quickly as possible, keep your knee straight and kick your right leg out behind you. Now, quickly, snap your leg back to the starting position. Repeat with your left leg. Exercise each leg five times, and progress as tolerated.

4 CRAWL KICK (for the backs of your legs and your buttocks)

Using a float, or holding onto the side of the pool, keep your knees straight and crawl kick. You want your heels to break the surface and make a lot of foam, but remember to keep your knees locked.

5 SIDE STEP (good for the outer thigh)

In shallow water, leading with your right leg, and keeping your knees straight, step as quickly as possible sideways. When you reach the side of the pool, lead with your left leg and return to starting place. Repeat five times. Progress by increasing the speed of your movement, and by increasing the depth of the water.

6 THE SIDELINER (to tone up the muscles of your waist and lower rib cage)

Stand with your back to the side of the pool and rest your arms on the edge for support. The water should be about the level of your armpits. Hold on tight now, and keep your leg straight. Bending from the waist, swing your legs as quickly as possible sideways. Quickly return to starting position, and swing them to the other side. Repeat five times for each side. Progress by increasing your speed and the number of times you do the exercise, as tolerated.

7 DOUBLE LEG LIFT

Note: This is the only place you should ever attempt to raise both legs at the same time, *never* on dry land. It is a strenuous abdominal exercise; doing it out of the water could injure your back.

Stand in chest-deep water with your back to the side of the pool, and use your arms to grip the edge for support. Make certain that you round your back before you begin the exercise by bending your knees very slightly. Now, tightening your stomach muscles, raise both legs as quickly as you can. Let them sink slowly to the starting position. Repeat the exercise five times. When you are sure your abdominal muscles are strong enough, keep your knees straight to perform the exercise. Progress by increasing the speed of the exercise, and increasing the number of times you perform it.

8 ARM CIRCLING (good for the upper arm)

Standing in water that is shoulder-high, quickly circle your arms backward twenty-five times. Reverse direction, and circle forward the same number of times.

9 SIDE ARM RAISE (for the upper arm and shoulders)

Standing in water that is shoulder-high, begin with both arms at your sides. Quickly raise them out to the sides so they are shoulder-level. Now quickly snap them back to your sides. Repeat five times and progress by increasing the speed of your movement, and the number of times you do the exercise.

16 About Face

At various times in my practice of physiotherapy, I have been asked to set up a programme of facial exercises designed to ward off, as long as possible, the inevitable wrinkles of time. There are, I know, several books on the subject, as well as a few private parlours where one can grimace away in secret.

Although I have been unable to find any statistics to substantiate the validity of facial exercises, or for that matter, statistics to prove they are invalid, it has been my experience that exercises of the facial muscles are of no practical value in slowing down the apparent aging process.

On the other hand, I have worked with patients suffering from partial paralysis of the facial muscles; the affected side is amazingly free of wrinkles and youthfully smooth. Similarly, I have worked with patients suffering from Parkinson's disease, people who have lost the quick use of their facial muscles, as well as other muscles throughout the body. There is a characteristic 'mask' ascribed to Parkinson victims because their faces lack expression, and thus are lacking lines even in old age. It would seem then that relaxation, or lack of use of the facial muscles – and not exercise – retards the wrinkling process.

There are many varied factors which combine to give the appearance of aging skin. Heredity, exposure to the elements, everyday pressures or emotional strain, inherent physiological constitution, and many other components all affect how and when your face will begin to show lines.

Have a good look at your face in the mirror. Aren't your facial lines just where your muscles are working most? If you are a smiler, you've got laugh lines. If you're quick to anger, there is probably a vertical line carved between your eyebrows. But if you are expert at hiding your feelings, so that no one really knows what is going on behind that cool exterior, you may be unusually free of wrinkles.

Creams, moisturizers, massage, or any of the things that allow your face to feel good and relaxed, are probably the best approach to the problem of aging and drying skin. Learning to relax entirely and totally is also worthwhile. In all good conscience, I cannot recommend any facial exercises. Better than that, relax your features, feel easy, and do learn to love your laugh lines. They are what give your face character.

Part Two:
Sixteen Minutes to Keep Your Shape

Until now, you have been working on particular parts of your body, toning up those areas where *you* need it most. Your choice. Now, here is a simple once over programme to keep you in super condition.

The exercises in Part One concentrated on the musculo-skeletal system. They were designed to shape you up for that marvellous effect on your appearance. To be sure, if you were to do them faithfully, those exercises would also have some beneficial effect on your heart and lungs. But there are other exercises designed to achieve that goal more specifically. By their very nature, they make your body work hard all over, promoting fitness in every sense of the word.

Because these exercises are of a more general type than the ones you have done previously, you will find that they are the kind which bring all the large muscle groups into play. They are exercises which will help to keep all your muscles in tone because they use these large muscle groups. And because they demand more from your entire body, they help promote fitness in the medical sense.

Most doctors, when they consider fitness, are not directly concerned with your slender profile. Though a trim appearance may have been the major factor which motivated you to undertake an exercise programme, physicians are primarily interested in your cardiovascular and respiratory fitness. That is, how your heart, blood vessels and lungs respond when you are working or exercising hard. Doctors may be concerned with your appearance too, but more than that, they are interested in the capacity of your body to do work.

Dr Kenneth Cooper, in his book, *Aerobics*, introduced a new word to the lay public, a word which often intrudes when discussing fitness. Aerobic power represents the oxygen transportation system. It is an index of how the body uses the oxygen which is available to it. Developing your cardiovascular fitness naturally helps to improve the body's use of oxygen, and that is exactly what the exercises in this chapter are designed to do. And while you are performing these exercises, they have the additional advantage of maintaining the muscle tone you have been working so hard to develop. This sixteen-minute programme then achieves success in two areas : (1) As a general maintenance programme for your best appearance. (2) To develop cardiovascular and respiratory fitness and thus better health.

Many of the exercises are similar to the type you find in the usual callisthenics class but for one essential difference. Here, we have eliminated the dangerous ones.

When you do these exercises properly, you will notice that your heart rate speeds up to approximately 130–150 beats per minute, that you are puffing when they are completed, and that you are probably perspiring. They should not be performed after a heavy meal, nor should they be done indiscriminately. That means that you should know that you are in good health before you begin. If you are under thirty and in good condition, you can probably undertake such a programme quite safely. If you are over thirty, or have any question about your general condition, do check with your doctor before you begin this or any other fitness programme. Saying this is not meant to frighten you. Rather, it is meant to assure you that you are going about this whole fitness routine in the best, safest, and easiest way possible. No professional worthy of his degree would suggest that you do otherwise – it is simply foolhardy !

Your physician will want to do some testing. First he will check your heart rate at rest, then again during and after exercise. By using a simple formula which considers your age and sex, he will then be in a position to tell you what heart rate is best for you to reach while exercising. Then he will show you how to monitor your own heart rate so that you can adjust or increase the time period for your exercise programme as you progress. In this way, the programme is individualized to suit you exactly.

As your fitness improves, you will continue to do the same exercises but increase the length of time you perform them to achieve the desired rate.

The programme includes four minutes of warm-up exercises, eight minutes of exercise to improve the efficiency and capacity of your heart, blood vessels and lungs, and four minutes of general conditioning exercises. You therefore begin with a sixteen-minute programme and increase the length of time when your heart rate is not raised sufficiently by exercising for that period. Exercising in this way, just three or four times a week, should keep you in super condition.

Part One
Four minutes (progress to eight depending on fitness level)

1 TWO ARM CIRCLING

Sitting on floor cross legged, arms outstretched, circle arms forward, then reverse.

2 LEG CIRCLING

Sitting on floor, legs outstretched, keep right knee locked and circle right leg first one way, then the other. Repeat with left leg.

3 HALF KNEE BEND

Standing with hands on hips, bend knees halfway. Then straighten knees and move up on your toes. Return to starting position. Repeat rapidly.

4 STANDING CALF STRETCH

Stand with a wide base and reach hands out in front of you. Keeping back straight, not rounded, bend forward and bounce slowly, feeling the pull behind your knees. (Not for someone with a bad back !)

5 KNEE TO FOREHEAD

In standing position, lift one knee as high as possible and bend to touch with forehead. Repeat with other knee. Repeat.

Part Two
Eight minutes (progress to fourteen minutes as fitness improves)

6 RUNNING ON THE SPOT: One minute to start.

7 LUNGE HOPS

Stand with one leg well in front of the other, the front knee bent. Hop to change legs. Repeat. Two minutes to start.

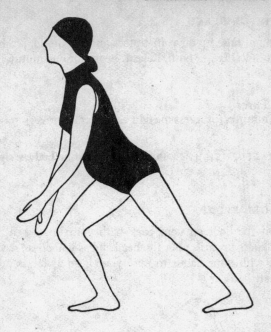

8 HIGH STEPPING

Use a sturdy table, stool or box 10 to 14 inches high. Step up with both feet and then down quickly, continuing for ten seconds. Rest for ten seconds. Repeat. Continue this for two minutes. Increase to three minutes as tolerated. As you improve, decrease the rest periods until you are able to keep stepping up steadily for three minutes.

9 SKIPPING: Using a skipping rope, skip slowly. For two minutes.

10 TIPTOE REACH

Standing, raise up on your tiptoes and as you do, reach arms out to sides. Lower both. Repeat. Begin for one minute.

Part Three
Four minutes (progress to eight as fitness improves)

11 HALF PUSH-UPS: Push-ups with your body weight on knees.

12 ROLL SIT-UP

Lie on the floor on your back with your knees bent. Raise both knees towards your forehead and as you do so, reach forward with your hands to raise your head as far as possible. Repeat.

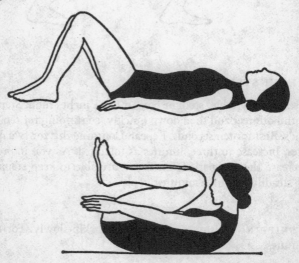

13 SIDE LEG CIRCLING

Lie on your left side and keeping your right knee straight, lift the leg a few inches and circle first one way and then the other. Change sides and repeat for left leg.

14 TENSION RELAXATION

Lie flat on your back and beginning with your feet tighten each muscle group all the way up your body. (Remember to bend your ankles up so your toes point to the ceiling to prevent foot cramping.) Include your calves, knees, stomach, buttocks, shoulders, arms and so on, all the way up, until your entire body is rigid. Hold for a count of five and then relax totally. Repeat twice more and rest in place.

Part Three:
Pre-Natal Care

18 What to Do until the Baby is Born

'So you're going to have a baby!' By this time, no matter what stage of pregnancy you are in, you have probably heard that phrase so often that you're considering setting it to music. It's a thrilling and exciting time, and while you share in all the excitement, you start to wonder if you should begin to take this whole thing seriously. After all, you *are* going to have a baby – your doctor told you so!

Among all the preparations for the baby's arrival – thinking of names, searching for cots, figuring out how many dozen nappies it will use a day – you may also have a small niggling question in the back of your mind: shouldn't you be doing something for *you*?

Well, there *are* some things you should be doing for you. And if you care enough about this wonderful new human being who is about to join your life, you'll make certain that its immediate environment is as perfect as you are able to make it. At present, that immediate environment happens to be you.

Why bother exercising now that you're pregnant? You're getting fatter anyway, you're really too tired, and besides, somebody told you not to strain yourself. Right? Wrong!

Follow a pre-natal programme because it does make a difference. You will feel better for it, before and after your pregnancy, and you will look better for it. Looking after yourself, keeping your body in the best possible condition, is a desirable goal at any time. Following a carefully planned rest and exercise programme during pregnancy is just as important to you and your baby as making sure you are eating properly. So let's talk about a good pre-natal programme, one that's safe, sensible, and realistic for you.

Basically, this programme is designed with three main aims in mind:

(1) To help you relax. That means that you will sleep better, and hence feel better, because you will get the full benefit from your rest. You will also be more comfortable during your labour.

(2) To tone up your muscles. It's important to you and the baby to keep your muscles in good shape at this time, and to avoid any unnecessary strain on your body in general, your back in particular.

(3) To help condition your body for this olympic activity in which you are about to become the star player. Labour is a strenuous and potentially exhausting activity; the better shape you are in, the more comfortable you will be before, during, and after.

Before we get into all the details, let's talk a bit about your anatomy so that we have a clearer understanding of the mechanics involved.

When you stand in an upright position, there is a normal low back curve, and that's just fine. As your baby grows, and your abdomen gets progressively bigger and heavier, you are literally thrown off balance. It's not quite the same as just suddenly gaining too much weight all over your body. In pregnancy, the weight gain is fairly well localized, mostly low and in front of you. In order to maintain your balance you lean backwards. When you do that, you are actually increasing the low back curve which puts a tremendous strain on the small muscles of the lower back. Muscles which are under excessive strain characteristically respond by going into spasm, and that hurts !

Now, it isn't a guarantee of pregnancy that you're in for your share of back aches, but it is fairly common, and that's the reason for exercising.

There are several things you can do to relieve the strain on your lower back. Doing them habitually will help you avoid the age-old problem of the ache if you haven't got it, or give you heaven-sent relief if you have.

Remember, if you increase the low back curve, you place extra strain on your muscles. If you flatten the curve out, you are offering relief to the small muscles of your lower back.

What you do from day to day counts. If you're the usual breed of housewife, you do most of your vacuuming and sweeping chores yourself. You take a broad-based stance when wielding a mop or broom, lean forward from the waist, and go to it. Don't! We've just been talking about the small muscles of your lower back which are under increased strain during pregnancy. When you lean forward from the waist, you are asking them to lift your entire torso, plus the added weight of the baby, and that is asking too much. You can bet those muscles will have something to say in protest by the time you're through.

When you have to vacuum, sweep, or whatever, place one foot in front of the other, keep your back straight, and rock back and forth on your feet to cover the area. If you must get down low, then do it the right way. Get on your knees or squat. Either way, you're saving your back.

How about those times when you can't move around? Perhaps you're standing at the stove, or doing the dishes, and you wish you knew how to make yourself more comfortable. Well, there is an easy and effective remedy for that one. Keep a low stool handy and rest one foot on it. When you do that, you automatically tilt your pelvis backwards and flatten out the low back curve, which, in turn, reduces the strain. You

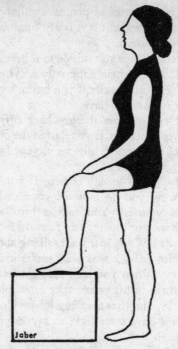

may just thank me for that one after a hard day over a hot stove.

What about the other chores that need to be done? Getting around on your hands and knees, believe it or not, is a healthy manoeuvre for the lady-in-waiting. When you stand erect, your abdominal organs and the baby you carry are under the influence of gravity and tend to fall down, pressing on the great veins, arteries, and nerves which pass through the pelvic cavity. On your hands and knees you relieve this situation temporarily and will probably feel better for it. Why not do your dusting and polishing that way then?

Carrying parcels is another fact of life that's hard to avoid.

If you're obviously pregnant, cultivating a helpless look is a good way to get eager hands and strong backs to your service. Or it may simply be a matter of smiling sweetly at some masculine type who will jump to the rescue. If you can manage to avoid the shopping altogether and have your husband do it for you, all well and good, but if he cannot, there are still a few things you can do to save your back.

Try to take your shopping in small doses. Not only do you have that lovely psychological advantage of having smaller bills to pay, but you also have smaller parcels to cart home.

A good idea is to divide the load and put the stuff into two shopping bags. That way, the weight is more evenly distributed and you're not forced to stagger home bags abreast. It's also easier on the back, keeping the weight down low.

If you find you're really stuck and must do a large shopping alone, take a shopping bag on wheels along and have the check-out girl fill it for you. Ask her to pack all the canned goods together and put them at the bottom of the bag. They won't spoil, and you can wait for someone else to give you a hand bringing them in.

There are lots of stores that deliver, and though you may want to choose your own meat and produce, it's a good thought to order your canned goods via the phone. They make up the heaviest portion of the load anyway.

Small parcels should be carried low and close, keeping them near your centre of gravity. The point is, although you may be healthier than you've ever been, you should be taking some precautions in caring for your back. That doesn't really mean pampering yourself unnecessarily, it means using common sense, and asking for help when something is too heavy for you to lift or carry. Remember, too, that when bending down to pick up a weight, your back should be straight and your knees bent. Your legs were built for carrying weight, so use them.

Sitting. How many times have you walked into a room, looked around for just the right place to sit, and chosen that lovely overstuffed comfy-looking thing that looks like you could live in it forever? Maybe you will! When the time comes to get up, you can't! If you do succeed in getting all of you out of all of it, at best you haven't done it gracefully. At worst you've strained your back.

The secret in choosing a good place to sit is to select a spot that doesn't look too comfortable. You want a chair with a firm back, and a slightly padded but solid seat. That's the sort of chair that will give you the best support and doesn't clutch onto you when it's time to leave.

Getting up gracefully is easy and a great back-saver, once you learn the rules. Shift forward on your seat until you feel that your bottom is quite near the edge. Put one foot back under the chair for added balance, and using your legs, keep your back straight and up you come. Simple as that.

This may come as a shocker, but for the lady-in-waiting, sitting with one leg crossed over the other is a no-no. When you are pregnant, the baby presses on the large veins that pass through the pelvic cavity on their way to the heart. These veins have a more difficult job than usual returning the blood to the heart due to the added load of the pregnancy itself. When you cross your legs at the knees, you are actually putting extra strain on them, and cramping them too. It just isn't fair. As a result, you may notice your ankles swelling, or your legs falling asleep, more often than usual.

So when you plunk yourself down for a rest, make it a whole body rest, and uncross your legs. You may, if you wish, cross them at the ankles or even slouch down in your chair if you like. But no crossed knees, please.

Another way to sit, although it may sound strange, is to squat. That is, with your feet parallel and about eighteen inches apart, crouch right down on your haunches. Getting the hang of it may be difficult at first, so you might want to begin practising while wearing a two-inch heel until you can balance yourself easily. You can then squat without shoes.

In primitive societies, women use the squatting position as the most comfortable and easiest way to deliver their babies. Not too long ago, delivery chairs were used so that something close to the squatting position was maintained. Today we use a delivery table and a modified squatting position as the feet are lifted and supported in stirrups. To accustom yourself to this position and allow you to be more comfortable while you're in it, practising squatting during your pregnancy is a good idea. When you have some potatoes to peel, or a telephone call to make, or just some time to read, try making good use of the time and squat.

Planning a long trip by car or plane is an exciting prospect, but you'll want to check with your doctor about the advisability of travelling at this time. All things being equal, your physician will probably tell you to go ahead and have a happy time. (That bumpy road nonsense is a thing of the past.)

Travelling by car can be fun, but plan to allow a little extra time to get where you're going. Frequent rest stops will likely be necessary, but don't just stop for a few moments to use the facilities. Plan to stop about once an hour and trot around the car a few times. It's good for the circulation, and will keep your legs from getting cramps or swelling. Bucket seats, you know, are so marvellously designed to cushion your rear that they get you right behind the knees. Nerves and blood vessels pass through that part of the leg fairly close to the surface, and the pregnant lady may find her legs becoming quite achy or swollen from the pressure of the seats. Exercising your legs often will be of help. Another tip is to put a small case in front of you so that you can rest your feet on it if you wish, and relieve the pressure of the bucket.

*

Rest is best. Having a good old-fashioned snooze at some point during the day can be a great reviver; when you're pregnant, it's an absolute must.

After coming home from a hard day over a typewriter, the usual procedure is to rush madly to the kitchen, do your best to prepare some semblance of a meal for hungry hubby. Then try not to nod off into your soup. Comes the struggle to clean up the clutter, drown the dishes, and shuffle off into the darkness.

If you're still working, and plan to continue as long as possible, you won't convince the boss that you're totally indispensable by lying down on top of your desk during the lunch break. But you still do need a rest, and I'm talking about the shades-drawn lights-out shoes-off kind. A working girl can fit that into her day if she plans right, and gets a little cooperation.

Warn your husband that dinner will be one hour later than usual – you won't be eating, you'll be dining! Then come home after work, turn off and tune out for one good hour's rest (you may want to set an alarm clock, or even better, have hubby wake you gently when he comes home). A nap before dinner, and you'll probably find that you're still capable of being good company for an evening, a pleasant surprise for both of you. Dinner will be later, it's true, but you and he will be happier for it.

If your day is really your own, and you can schedule your time as you like, the optimum time for a rest is mid-day. Have it around noon if you plan to lunch out with the ladies, or, better still, after the luncheon meal if you can fit it in. You'll honestly find you feel better, really refreshed.

Better safe. You would be well advised to read the section, *Safe and Sound,* found in Chapter One. If it sounds reasonable to take simple precautions for your safety when you're not pregnant, how much more important it is to you now that you are. Why take the risk of unnecessary injury to you or the baby? Let's face it, no matter how feminine you are feeling, you're just not quite as light on your feet as you used to be. It will pay to be extra careful.

Underneath it all? Selecting maternity clothes can now be a full-time occupation for the fashion-conscious. The needle trade has finally recognized that there is an ever-growing market in expectant mothers, and a whole new industry has blossomed, dedicated to the lady-in-waiting. The case for the vanishing waistline has assumed great new proportions. But just as you can now choose from infinite racks of bathing suits, jeans, and fabulous formals, you also find yourself confronted with a whole new series of weird-looking underthings. It just might help to know what you really need before you get caught in the underworld.

Breast tissue is not elastic, it is made up mostly of glandular and fatty tissue. (I've gone into some detail about this in Part One, Chapter Six, and it would be well worth your while to read up on it now.) Tissue which is not muscular, that is, non-elastic, does not snap back into shape after being stretched, and that's an important point to remember if you're pregnant.

At this time in your life, your breasts may achieve such proportions you may marvel that you had it in you. The glands are enlarging in preparation for the production of milk, and there is some increase in fatty tisue as well. In all, you may easily gain two pounds in the bosom alone.

If you don't want to chance sagging breasts after the birth of your baby, it's most important that you support them well now, while they are heavy.

A common mistake is to buy your regular bra in a larger size. Don't do it. The average bra just doesn't have the kind of support we're talking about. You need a good maternity bra for adequate support. Here's a timely tip: In the latter part of your pregnancy, your breasts are as large as they are going to get, even if you plan to nurse. When you are nursing your baby, the breasts get heavier but not bigger in size. So if you do plan to breast feed, you can save yourself the trouble and expense of shopping for underwear twice, by buying and wearing your nursing bras before the baby comes. A good nursing bra has all the support you may need, and it's comfortable too.

Thank heavens the era of the round garter is long past. Those awful bits of elastic practically guaranteed varicose veins by impeding the blood flow from the legs back to the heart. If you were lucky enough to escape those unsightly blue maps, aching legs and swollen ankles were the order of the day. But most women don't wear garters today, so why do I bother to mention them? Because we have a few things to learn from the mistakes of the past.

Don't wear any kind of constricting garments, especially around your legs. We don't need garters today because we have stockings that stay up, all by themselves. But it's a good bet that if they're tight enough to stay up, they're too tight. The same goes for knee-high stockings. If they ridge your flesh, forget them. You're far better off buying one of those crazy maternity garter belts that sling over the shoulders, or investing in maternity pantyhose even though they cost a little more. The price you may have to pay for impeding the circulation in your legs is really too high.

What about a maternity girdle? Any self-respecting maternity shop would consider itself a shameful failure if it didn't try to sell you one. A sale may be good for business, but it's not good for you. Unless your back is so bad that your doctor insists on one of these contraptions for the little extra support it may provide, do yourself a favour and save your shape. The problem with these two-way terrors is that they hold your stomach in for you; they do the work your abdominal muscles should be doing. The results are disastrous. Your abdominals, like all other muscles that are not being worked, lose their shape and tone. Combine this with the normal stretching due to pregnancy, and when it's all over you're in bad shape.

Keep it up. A common complaint of pregnancy is swollen legs. You will usually notice this swelling after being on your feet for some time, or during warm weather. If so, get your feet up. I mean really up, the higher the better.

The pressure of the baby on the blood vessels which pass through the pelvic cavity does put some extra strain on the circulation. The combined effect of this and gravity is a tendency to pooling of the blood in the legs. Raising the legs, then, counteracts this tendency. When you're sitting, rest your legs as high as you can. In bed, use a couple of extra pillows under your legs to keep them up. If you really want effective relief, get your legs up higher than your heart. A good way to do that is the right-angle position. Lie on your back on the floor and rest your legs up on the wall. It works beautifully.

If you should notice a sudden swelling of your hands and feet, and you find that you've gained a lot of weight in a very little time, do let your doctor know about it. He might want to check you over as a precaution. Although some swelling is to be expected, a lot of swelling could be an indication of something else, and your physician is the best judge of that.

Carrying it off is important. Good posture is important to your health and feeling of well-being when you're not pregnant, but so much more so when you are. It's hard to really look good when your back is killing you, but if your posture is good it may save you hours of aches and pains.

The major muscle groups which help you to stand erect are

called the antigravity muscles. When your posture is correct, these muscles work with a maximum of efficiency and minimum of effort. The increasing size and weight of your stomach actually tend to throw you off balance when you are pregnant, and to put an unaccustomed strain on the antigravity muscles, particularly those of the back. If your abdominal muscles are weakened, and not supporting the uterus as well as they might, this increases the strain and usually results in the typical back ache of pregnancy. Correcting poor posture in pregnancy is simply a matter of learning how, and improving the condition and tone of your abdominal muscles, all of which reduces the strain on the lower back.

The pelvis is the bony girdle around which good posture is built. When you relax your abdominal muscles, or let it all

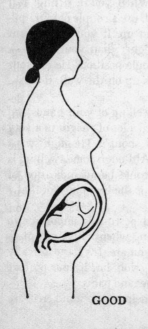
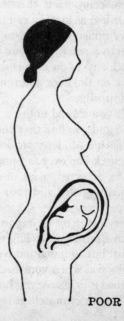

GOOD   POOR

hang out, the pelvis tilts forward and allows the baby to lean out of this bony cradle, effectively using the abdominal muscles like a hammock and stretching them unnecessarily. When you pull in your stomach, you tilt the pelvis backward, that is, tuck your buttocks under, and the baby is then properly supported in the pelvis with less strain on you. In this position then, the muscles of your front and back are perfectly balanced, and there goes the back ache.

Try standing in front of a mirror and correcting your posture. Stand with your feet three or four inches apart, and your back straight. Now pull in your stomach and tuck your tail under. Don't be discouraged if you have difficulty achieving this at first. When you begin to practise pelvic tilting as part of the exercise programme, it will come more easily. Correct your posture as often as you think of it; it will be well worth the effort.

Eating for two? You're feeling terrific; you've got that pregnant glow; you're forever famished – and your doctor tells you to put your appetite in the deep freeze. Whatever happened to the old myth about eating for two? It's been debunked! Calorifically speaking, you're still eating for you, and if you don't, you're going to find you're a big fat mamma when it's all over. Nutritionally, however, the value of the food you eat during your pregnancy should go away up.

Your diet during pregnancy plays a major role in the development of your unborn child, and you will probably want to discuss it with your doctor. He can tell you what you should be including or excluding, and whether your eating habits, as they stand, make for a well-balanced diet. But there are a few tips I can give you that you may find helpful.

At some time during your pregnancy, your doctor will probably tell you to put the lid on the cookie jar – that is, don't gain too much weight. (How much is too much is up to your own doctor.) But now is not the time to go off on some crazy fad diet. They're not terrific at any time (few of them are properly balanced), but when you're pregnant they're out. Still, there are a few things you can do to help keep the scale from blowing its top.

Get rid of the 'empty-calorie' foods around you. That's the nibble stuff, things like 'chips' and 'cheezies'. Don't even have them in the house, and the temptation just won't be there. If you must nibble, keep some celery or carrot sticks handy. Not only are they low in calories, but the chewing makes you feel like you're really eating something, and they have some nutritional value too. Instead of eating canned fruits, eat raw. Again, the chewing fools you into thinking you've had a bigger portion, and the number of calories you're downing is cut tremendously. Not all fruits are low in calories, however, and you'll want to keep a calorie counter handy to check them out. (You'll be amazed at how many calories there are in a slice of watermelon!)

Take some extra care to see that the meat you choose is lean. Substituting with fish and poultry is even better. You get the same food value with lower calories, and a larger portion for a comparable weight. Remember that your protein needs during pregnancy increase by half, so you need meat, fish, and poultry in your diet.

Try to include a salad with your meals: lots of extra chewing, a good filler, low in calories. A salad may also give you the happy bonus of helping overcome the constipation so common in pregnancy.

At some point, your doctor will probably tell you to cut down on your salt intake. If he tells you to cut it out completely, you'll want him to explain to you just how far he wants you to go. But if it's just a matter of excluding extra salt from your diet, here are a few tips you may find helpful.

Chemically, salt is sodium chloride. It is the sodium part of the name that you have to watch out for, and avoid. Anything, then, that has salt or sodium as part of its name is not for you. That includes such condiments as garlic salt, onion salt, and so on, some of which have substitute powders you can use in your cooking. Most of the good old bubbly remedies for indigestion, you will find, contain some form of salts and as a result, are included on your 'no' list. Baking soda, too, is another big offender.

There are a few foods that by their very nature are high in salt content, and you should be aware of them. Smoked meats and fishes contain large amounts of salts used in the curing process. Eating your fill of Chinese delicacies, food which is liberally laced with monosodium glutamate, is tantamount to downing a glass of salt water.

You can find a salt substitute on the market but it hardly seems worth the effort. Cultivating a taste for it really takes some doing, and it's just a matter of time until that baby comes and you may again include salt as a regular part of your diet.

The problem with salt, you see, is that it produces the tendency for water retention. Voilà, the swollen ankles so common in pregnant women. Swelling of the hands and feet is an annoyance and decidedly uncomfortable, it's true, but worse, it can lead to complications you'd rather avoid. Your doctor may prescribe a diuretic, or water pill, if he feels you need it.

What pregnant woman has not, at some time during her pregnancy, experienced heartburn? Sometimes even water seems to bring it on. Aside from the dubious honour of producing a hairy-chested infant – so the superstition goes ! – no one really wants to suffer from that unpleasant burning sensation. You will quickly discover those foods which are your worst enemies, and the best solution is simply to eliminate them from your diet. Some women find fried foods or highly spiced dishes give them the most trouble. Others complain about gassy vegetables like cucumber or cabbage. Eliminate those foods which are the worst offenders for you.

If heartburn really seems to plague you no matter what you eat, you may find it decreased by drinking a glass of milk before meals. This tends to coat the stomach. Another way to fight the fire is to divide your three large meals of the day into six small meals. That is, eat the same total amount as you are used to doing, but eat smaller quantities at each sitting, and eat more often.

Remember, baking soda as a remedy is out, but you will probably find that the antacid you buy over the counter is a life saver.

During your pregnancy the foundation of your baby's body, its bones, are being built. Milk and milk products are still the best source of calcium even though you may be taking calcium pills as a safeguard. If you can't face a glass of milk even on your best days, an ounce of cheese gives you about the same amount of calcium as a glass of milk, so you can substitute that way. If cheese turns you off too, talk to your doctor about it; he may recommend an alternative.

A well-balanced diet includes sufficient amounts of carbohydrates, vitamins, minerals, proteins, and other dietary necessities. You will likely be taking iron pills and vitamins prescribed by your doctor as a supplement, but he still prefers that you get all these good things from your food. If you are not sure that your diet is, in fact, well-balanced, or have some questions about the kind of foods you are eating, don't hesitate to discuss this with your doctor or a professional dietitian. They are your best sources of guidance, and can help you work out an eating plan that is sensible and tailored to meet your own individual needs.

One last pointer about the food you eat: don't be carried away by a new report in your favourite magazine or newspaper. Most often these stories make good print but are incomplete, incorrect, or simply misleading. Remember, too, that the total weight of baby plus associated pregnancy weight will be approximately fourteen pounds; all the rest you gain is you.

19 Pre-Natal Exercises

Being prepared now, to you, means getting yourself physically and mentally ready for the labour and delivery of your baby.

The exercise programme may be started any time after your third month of pregnancy has passed. You will find it is divided into four lessons. All of the exercises are medically safe and effective for pregnant women, and unless your doctor has specifically told you not to exercise, you will find this programme of tremendous value. If you are unable to do the suggested number of exercises, do as many as you can. Your muscles will improve with working, and you will soon find you can do them all. None of these exercises should cause you any pain. If you find that one does, eliminate it for the time being. You are probably doing it wrong, so wait until your next doctor's appointment, and have him check you out on it.

Start your programme by doing Lesson One for one week. Do each exercise five times, and the entire programme at least once a day – twice is better if you have the time. After a week, add on the exercises of Lesson Two, and do both lessons for a week. Progress in this manner until you are doing all four lessons, and then continue to do these exercises *at least* once daily until the birth of your baby.

Lesson One

1 SHOULDER CIRCLING (a good warm-up exercise, also helps to loosen the upper back)

With your hands on your shoulders, slowly make nice big circles with your arms. Make twenty-five circles going clockwise, then reverse direction and repeat.

2 FOOT CIRCLING (another warm-up, good for improving circulation in the legs. Do this at the beginning of each exercise session; do it if your legs are particularly bothersome or swollen; and remember to do it as soon as you can after the baby is born.)

Sitting on the floor with your legs straight out in front of you, begin by making slow circles with your right foot. Allow your leg to rest on the floor as you do this, but remember to keep your knee straight. Go around twenty-five times, then reverse direction. Repeat the exercise with your left foot.

3 PELVIC TILT (This is a great exercise for preventing the low back ache so common in pregnancy, or for relieving the discomfort if you already have it. At the same time, it strengthens the abdominal muscles.)

Lie on the floor with your knees bent so that your feet are flat on the floor. Slip your hand under the small of your back and feel a slight hollow. Now tighten your stomach muscles, and press your back down into your hand so that you are rounding your back. Now that you've got the idea, remove your hand and repeat the exercise. Hold the contraction for the count of five, then relax. Repeat five times. (See diagram p. 146.)

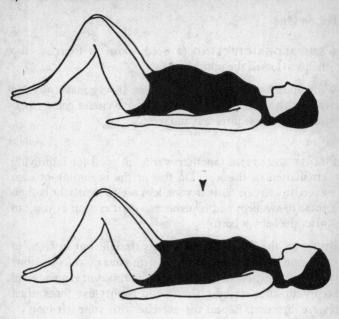

4 HEAD AND SHOULDER RAISE (strictly an abdominal exercise)

Lie on your back with your knees bent, and your feet flat on the floor. Lift your head and shoulders up off the floor, as you reach with both hands towards your knees. Hold it there for the count of five. Lower slowly. Repeat five times.

5 REACH ACROSS (an abdominal exercise which works on the diagonal abdominal muscles)

Lie on your back with your knees bent and your feet flat on the floor. With your right hand, reach to the outside of your left knee. Hold for a count of five and lower slowly. Now reach with your left hand to the outside of your right knee. Hold and relax. Repeat five times.

6 HUMPING AND HOLLOWING (works on your stomach and back)

Get up on your hands and knees so that your hands are under your shoulders. Lower your head and tuck your chin in as

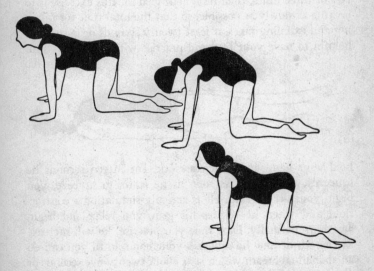

you slowly round your back like a cat. Now, very slowly, look up towards the ceiling, and as you do, arch your back. Repeat five times.

7 ABDOMINAL BREATHING (This is one type of breathing which will be used during your labour; though it may not

seem natural at first, practice will make it come easily and comfortably. It is helpful to do this one in bed.)

Lie on your back, well-supported with pillows, if you wish. Put one hand on the bulge of your stomach to help you as you practise. Quickly and sharply blow out the air you have in your lungs, but don't waste time doing it. Now, very slowly, breathe in through your nose, and as you do so, make your stomach rise. When you have reached the limit of your capacity, exhale slowly through your mouth. Practise this two or three times, then rest. Your goal for this exercise is to breathe as slowly as possible, so that the total time for inhaling and exhaling takes at least twenty seconds or more. It is helpful to have your husband practise with you. Have him

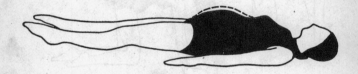

hold your hand and watch a clock. For fifteen seconds he squeezes your hand. As soon as he starts to squeeze, you begin your deep breath. He is actually simulating a contraction, and when he relaxes his grip, you relax and begin breathing normally. Each time you practise, he will increase the length of time he squeezes your hand, until you can do an abdominal breath which lasts about twenty-five seconds or more. Remember, at no time do you hold your breath. Breathing as slowly as you can, you are aiming to do only two breaths per minute with no holding between.

8 RELIEVING LEG CRAMPS (This isn't an exercise, but it's a trick you'll be excited to learn if you are one of so

many who are awakened during the night with an awful cramp in the calf of your leg.)

The usual method to relieve such a cramp is to try to massage it out. That takes time, it's agonizing, and it really doesn't work. This does. Have your husband grip the heel of the stricken leg in his hand and apply pressure to the forefoot with his forearm. At the same time he presses on your knee with his other hand to keep it straight. This stretches the calf muscle, and it is a physiological phenomenon that it will relax. In a moment the cramp is gone, I promise.

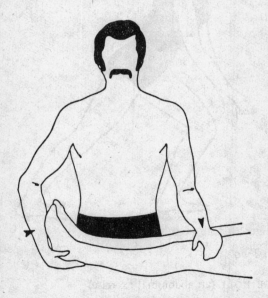

If you haven't got your husband handy, or he doesn't respond very joyfully when he's awakened at three in the morning, there is another way to get rid of the cramp, but it's not as much fun. Get out of bed and stand up. Place the cramped leg behind you, keeping your knee straight and your foot pointed forward. Now lunge forward on your other leg and hold the position until the cramp passes.

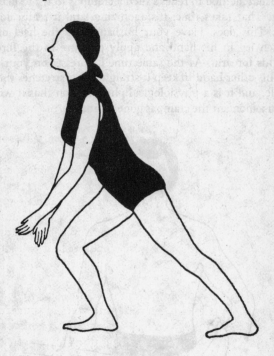

Lesson Two

1 KNEE ROLL (an abdominal exercise)

Lie on your back with your knees bent and your feet flat on the floor. Very slowly lower both knees to the right. Slowly bring them back to mid-line and then over to the left. Repeat five times.

2 STRAIGHT LEG RAISE (good for the circulation; helps strengthen the leg muscles as well)

Lie on your back with your left knee bent and the foot flat on the floor. Tighten your right knee, keeping your leg straight, and lift your right leg about ten inches off the floor. Take the leg out to the right, then to the left, back to the centre and down. Repeat the exercise with your left leg. Relax. Repeat five times.

3 RELAXATION

There are many ways to learn relaxation, from self-hypnosis to stretching techniques. But I've found this method most helpful to pregnant women as it really demonstrates the difference in feeling between being tight and being relaxed. The first few times you try the technique, you may not feel any benefit, but with regular practice it can really do wonders. Not only will you be able to relax on command during your labour, but sleep will forever come easily if you learn to follow your own orders. It has the added bonus of being a great body toner too.

Beginning at your feet, and travelling up your body, tighten each muscle group in turn until you feel your muscles really straining. When you feel you can hold it no longer, let go, and feel your whole body relax as though you were on an air mattress floating gently on the sea. Start, then, by tightening your toes, bending your feet up at the ankles, tightening your knees, your buttocks and thighs. Stretch your legs and your back. Pull your shoulders back and straighten your arms. Clench your fists until your knuckles are white. Pull in your stomach and stretch your neck so your chin is pulled in. Hold it until you can't hold it any longer, then relax with a sigh and feel yourself float. Repeat at least three times, and always practise at least once before you go to sleep.

4 PANTING (This is another form of breathing you will be
   using during your labour. It may not seem easy at first, but
   a little practice will have you doing it easily.)

Panting is used in labour in two different ways. You will use
it during your contractions in combination with your abdominal breathing, and we will come to that in Lesson Three.
But there may be another time you need to pant. At some
point in your labour you will want to push because you have
the urge, but your doctor may tell you not to. It's tough not
to, when you feel you have to, but he may ask you not to
nevertheless. So what you do is pant. That takes the pressure
of the diaphragm off the uterus, and you no longer push. So
remember, if the man says 'Don't push' – pant.

   How to pant? Quite easy, really. Practise like this at first.
Sit in tailor sitting position with your legs crossed, and put
one hand on your stomach and one on your chest. It helps to
watch yourself in front of a mirror. Take quick shallow
breaths (like a dog panting in the summer heat) so that there
is no movement of your stomach, and the only movement
you feel is of your chest. Practise this for short periods at intervals during your exercise programme.

Lesson Three

1 PELVIC FLOOR EXERCISE

The muscles of the pelvic floor are the ones which surround
the urethra, the vaginal outlet, and the anus. These muscles
are tremendously stretched during delivery, but unlike com-
mercial elastic which when overworked loses elasticity,
muscle tissue becomes more elastic, or stretchable, with work
and exercise.

   Doing this exercise will also strengthen the muscles of the

vaginal wall which grip the penis during intercourse; it may therefore be one of the most important exercises you'll ever do !

The nice thing about this little exercise is that you can do it standing or sitting, while you're washing dishes or waiting for a bus, and no one will ever know.

Lie on your back with your legs out straight and crossed at the ankles. Squeeze your buttocks together and pull up between your legs as though you were trying to stop from passing your urine. (You can check to see if you've got the right method by actually stopping in mid-flow.) As you tighten the muscles, count to ten. Then relax. Repeat five times. Practise as often as you think of it during the day.

2 INNER THIGH STRETCH (Doing this exercise will help you to be more comfortable during the delivery, and it's an easy one to practise while watching television.)

Sit on the floor with the soles of your feet touching. Rest your elbows on your knees, and using the pressure of your body weight, rock on your knees trying to get them to touch the floor. You can feel the muscles of your inner thigh being stretched.

3 PUSHING

This is an urge which comes naturally near the end of your labour. It is much like trying to pass a difficult bowel movement, but it is directed forward. You really don't have to be taught how to do it because you'll know how when the time comes. I want to remind you, however, that you can mechanically aid the pushing by taking a deep breath and lifting your head when you are asked to push hard. This increases abdominal pressure and helps with the expulsion of the baby.

4 BREATHING

You've learned how to do abdominal breathing and how to pant. Now it's time to put them together as you would during a contraction. It's a good idea to practise with your husband who can keep his eye on the clock and make certain that you follow the routine, through the period of one minute.

Begin by quickly exhaling just to ready yourself for the deep breathing. Slowly inhale through your nose as much as you can, then exhale as slowly as possible through your mouth. When you have completed exhaling, do four or five short pants. Then do another abdominal breath, inhaling slowly through your nose, and breathing out slowly through your mouth. That routine should take you through the period of one minute. If it doesn't, practise often, trying to increase the time it takes you to do the routine.

Some women never do achieve the goal of doing only two abdominal breaths with the one period of panting between. If this is the case for you, you may add on another series of pants, and then one more abdominal breath. This is sure to carry you over the minute, which is the aim of the game. You want to be in complete control of your breathing during contractions, and know exactly what you are doing. So practise frequently and you will be comfortable and confident.

Lesson Four

You have been doing the pre-natal exercise programme for three weeks now, and are probably well on your way to feeling better and really getting into condition. We have covered all the exercises important to your programme, but there is one exercise we are now going to adjust, and that is relaxation.

From now on, when you practise relaxation, instead of contracting each muscle group of your entire body, you are going to contract only one, and use that as a signal to relax.

With your hands at your sides, press your hands into the bed as hard as you can. Hold it. Then relax. As you do so, feel the floating sensation as your whole body relaxes. Learn to distinguish the difference between feeling tight and feeling relaxed, so that during your labour, when a contraction has passed, you can say 'relax' to yourself, and really experience the feeling.

Pregnancy Chart

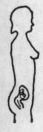

Third Month
Your abdomen and breasts grow larger. Your baby is in a 'floating' position, weighs about an ounce and is 3 inches long. His arms, legs and head are just distinguishable.

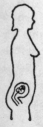

Fourth Month
Maternity clothes may be required by now. Your baby is now about 6 inches long and weighs ¼ lb. You may feel his first movements.

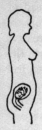

Fifth Month

The skin on your abdomen stretches considerably. The doctor can hear your baby's heartbeat with a stethoscope, and his movements are more easily felt. He is about 10 inches long and weight is about ½ lb.

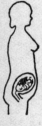

Sixth Month

As your abdomen continues to enlarge, your baby's movements become more vigorous. His skin is red, wrinkled and covered with soft down, and hair has begun to grow on his head. He is now about 12 inches long, weighing 1½ lbs.

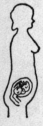

Seventh Month

Your baby's eyes are open. If he is born at this time, he has some chance of survival. He weighs about 2½ lbs. and is about 15 inches in length.

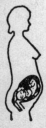

Eighth Month

Your baby's movements, more forceful, may be seen from outside. His weight has increased to about 4 lbs. and his length to about 16½ inches. His skin is not as wrinkled, and he is in the position in which he will be born (normally, head down).

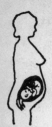

Ninth Month
Your baby settles lower into the
abdomen, ready for birth. Most of the
fuzzy down on his body has
disappeared, and his head may be
covered with hair. He weighs at least
6 or 7 lbs. and is about 20 inches or
more in length.

Reprinted from *My Baby Book* published by Wyeth Ltd, Toronto,
Ontario.

20 What to Do after the Baby is Born

You've actually done it! Produced a baby! You came through with flying colours. As you tear down the hall to the scales, you catch a glimpse of yourself in the mirror. It just can't be! You still look pregnant!

You may as well face it, those slender slacks you brought for the return trip are closer to baby's size than your own. You'll still have to wear your maternity dress, not at all what you had in mind.

Well, there's no reason why you really have to stand for that flabby figure for long, especially if you were smart enough to exercise during your pregnancy. The extra weight will drop off easily if you didn't break the scales with over-indulgence, and the inches will come off too. Having a baby, or two, or five, is no excuse for being out of shape. If you don't like the way you look, there's lots you can do about it.

As soon as your doctor gives you the cue, which should be shortly after the baby has arrived, you can begin your programme to become the sveltest mother on the block.

Here's a list of simple exercises to help you reach the goal — back into your pre-baby wardrobe by your six-week check-up or sooner. Do these exercises at first in bed, then on the floor, and begin by doing each five times daily. After five days, do them at least twice daily, and increase the number of repetitions until you can do them each twenty times.

1 BOOK PRESS

Lie on your back with your knees bent and your feet flat on the floor. Put a book between your knees and press your knees against the book. As you do so, tighten your stomach muscles and buttocks. Hold for a count of five. Relax. Repeat five times.

2 PELVIC TILT

Lie on your back with your knees bent and your feet flat on the floor. Slip your hand under your back and feel the slight hollow. Now tighten your stomach muscles and press your back down into your hand so that you round your back. Got the idea? Remove your hand and repeat. Hold for the count of five. Relax. Repeat five times.

3 KNEE ROLL

Lie on your back with your knees bent and your feet flat on the floor. Roll your knees slowly to the right, then slowly back to mid-line, and over to the left. Try to keep your torso still while you do this, and tighten your stomach muscles. Repeat five times.

4 PELVIC FLOOR EXERCISE

Lie flat on your back with your ankles crossed. Pull up between your legs as though you are trying to stop from passing your urine. As you do this, tighten your buttocks. Hold for the count of five and repeat five times.

5 TWO HAND REACH

Lie on your back with your knees bent and your feet flat on the floor. Lift your head up, and with both hands, reach towards your knees. Hold for the count of five. Lower slowly. Repeat five times.

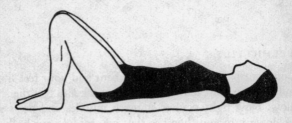

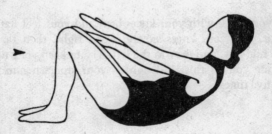

6 SIDE BEND

Lie flat on your back. Tighten your stomach muscles and slide your right hand down towards your right knee, bending sideways. Return to mid-line and repeat to the left. Repeat five times.

7 CROSS HAND REACH

Lie on your back with your knees bent and your feet flat on the floor. Lift your head, tighten your stomach muscles, and reach your right hand towards the outside of your left knee. Lower slowly. Then reach your left hand to the outside of your right knee. Repeat five times.

All the above exercises are specifically designed to work those muscles most likely to require toning after pregnancy. Doing them regularly should get you quickly back into good shape. If there's more you'd like to do, however, after your six-week check-up is a good time to set up a routine for yourself, using those exercises you want for your own individual needs, from the general chapters of this book. They're all safe and medically sound, and great shapers.

Part Four:
Post-Cardiac Care

21 What to Do after a Heart Attack

In North America alone, the number of heart attack victims reaches into the many thousands. If you are among them, if you have had a heart attack (myocardial infarction), you may have some adjustments to make in your activities. If all goes well, and your recovery is uneventful, there is no reason why you cannot return eventually to a normal productive life. Accepting that fact is the first step in reaching your objective.

If you have had a heart attack, your attitude about it will have a great deal to do with your ability to return to a life of activity and satisfaction. Feeling depressed or sorry for yourself will not help you in your recovery, it will only work against you. Knowing a little about heart disease and its effects, on the other hand, will probably help you to recognize your good fortune in having medical science on your side, and will enable you to look at things in a positive way.

There is no firm data to support the theory that a vigorous exercise programme retards the disease process, or prevents the recurrence of further attacks. There is, however, strong proof that a person who is physically fit is more able to withstand a heart attack. There is no doubt among medical authorities that exercise will make you more fit, and as such, you are in better condition to survive another attack should it occur. Psychologically too, exercise is invaluable in your rehabilitation programme. As you see yourself progress, you realize that you can return to a normal life and do most things everyone else does without detriment. You needn't become a cardiac cripple.

In my research it has become evident that variations in physical and psychological make-up, the differences in individual attacks, and the variations in the recovery period, make it necessary to treat each heart attack patient individually. There are conflicting opinions regarding the types of exercise thought to be beneficial. As a result, your programme *must* be based on what your doctor finds to be pertinent to your own individual needs. It is impossible to set up a programme that applies to everyone without inviting unnecessary danger. Don't let some fast-talking 'health club' operator try to convince you otherwise. Unless there are proper medical facilities immediately at hand, signing the contract may be the last thing you do.

Although the types of exercise thought best are still under controversy, it is generally agreed, according to leading cardiologists, that exercise, when properly monitored, does improve general well-being. There is no doubt that you improve your working capacity as the cardiovascular response to exercise improves. Exercise can and does delay the onset of angina, and it also increases the oxygen supply to the heart muscle.

Angina, or the fear of it, can disable one enough to impair function and the resumption of normal living. At a recent conference of cardiologists in the United States, it was generally agreed that with exercise, the threshold for angina improves, which allows the individual to function at a higher level. There is also evidence, they agreed, that people who exercise are in better condition to fight their illness. There is no evidence that exercise is at all harmful if properly supervised and adjusted to the individual.

Although exercise is thought to prolong longevity, there are no statistics available to substantiate this. Factors such as diet, emotional stability, and stresses of daily life have a direct bearing on your well-being and recovery. There may also be hereditary factors to consider. All these are elements on which your doctor can base his judgement regarding your suitability for an exercise programme.

It is generally agreed that no one who has suffered a heart attack should begin really exercising before three months have passed. Your body needs this time for scar tissue to form in the damaged tissue, and to allow the heart to recover. If there are no complications, and recovery runs an uneventful course, the American Heart Association has a few suggestions it considers prudent to follow.

Your doctor, before allowing you to begin an exercise programme, will want you to wait three months. He will then make certain that there is no congestive heart failure and that there are no abnormal beats at rest, during exercise, or during the recovery period after exercises have been performed. This he learns through a series of specific tests. You may have steady exertional angina, but should have none at rest or during the night. Also, you should not have a recently changed pattern of exertional angina, and your resting cardiogram must be stable.

It is important to remember, too, that any exercise programme will do you no good if you are not abiding by the other advice your physician offers. That is, you must stop smoking, and you must keep to a reasonable weight. If after adequate laboratory tests, and after testing the working capacity of your heart, your doctor advises that you would do well with an exercise programme, you must still use your common sense. If you become excessively tired, or experience any shortness of breath, or pain, *stop what you are doing*.

Ideally, all exercise programmes should be medically supervised. There is not adequate supervision at most of the so-called health clubs, and it is important that you understand the risk of exercising at such a place. To exercise without the benefits of monitoring devices, and without medical equipment on the spot, is pure folly. Any doctor worth his oath would advise against it.

It is clear, then, that an exercise programme for a person who has had a coronary attack must be totally individualized, as each patient has a unique problem. Limits will be set for you, and you must not exceed them. Your programme should be detailed as to the number of minutes you are to work. Usually the programme is designed to use the large muscle groups, and to increase endurance. Jogging, treadmill, and running are often the exercises of choice. Isometric exercises, and working with springs and weights, are absolutely out. Competitive sports and games are also excluded from your programme, as it is impossible to measure the dose of such exercise; it is all too easy to exceed your capacity when you are trying to win.

Since walking is good exercise, golf is a sport you may continue to play safely, as long as you avoid the hilly holes and don't lose your temper when you play. When betting is involved, however, the emotional strain may be more trying than the actual physical effort involved, so it's best to play just for fun. Remember, too, not to carry a heavy bag.

Activities which require sudden bursts of effort, such as tennis or running up stairs, should be avoided. If you are going to bowl, choose five- instead of ten-pin. Avoid vigorous armwork sports, such as canoeing and rowing. Remember, whatever you are doing, don't rush into it. Exercise in moderation.

Your exercise programme should include a warm-up period, a period of good exercise, and a cooling-off period as well. The intensity of the exercises must be high enough to get a stimulus, but not above your set limits. For those reasons, it is again important that you be checked during and after your exercises by a doctor, to make certain the programme is right for you.

While you and your doctor are considering the advisability of an exercise programme, you may also have questions about how you are to proceed in your activities of daily living.

Your emotions have an important effect on your state of health, and you would be wise to remember that. In other words, stay cool. If a problem should arise, at business or home, try to deal with it calmly and sensibly. If you can see you are having difficulty working it out, get help. Don't let your everyday worries get you down; it just isn't worth it. Use your common sense— everything in moderation.

Like your exercise programme, your daily activity should be similarly arranged. Allow yourself time in the morning to warm up to the day's activities. Don't rush right off to work after a big breakfast, but take a few minutes to digest your food. Work up gradually to a full day's activity, and at the end of the day slow down and cool off.

Rest is important to you. You should strive for moderation in your sleeping habits. Staying up late one night, and trying to catch up the next, is not the best arrangement. You should try to get about the same amount of rest each night, even if it means resting before you go out for what you expect will be a late evening. Resting during the day is also advisable. If you have a hobby, or an activity you find particularly restful, you may want to include it in your day as part of your resting time.

Because extreme heat and cold put extra strain on the heart, they should be avoided. That means it is important to dress appropriately for the weather, so that you will not be overheated or very cold. On a cold day, wrapping a scarf around your face is a good idea so that you don't take deep breaths of cold air. Snow shovelling, of course, is out, since it is a strenuous activity which requires sudden bursts of energy combined with exposure to cold weather. When it is very hot and humid, don't overdo it. Dress comfortably and try to stay cool. Saunas, of course, are to be avoided.

Keeping to a reasonable weight is essential to your health. When you are overweight, your heart is under additional strain. Do not overeat at any one meal. Divide your daily food intake into three or four well-balanced meals. Rest after eating to allow sufficient time for digestion; any strenuous activity immediately after eating poses an unnecessary strain on your heart.

Remember that caffeine is a stimulant; eliminating coffee from your diet makes good sense. There are many good brands of caffeine-free coffee now on the market, so why not choose one as a safe substitute? Tea and some colas also contain caffeine, so take them in moderation.

Since alcohol is also a drug, and everyone reacts differently to it, ask your doctor how much you can drink safely.

Diet fads, and articles on nutrition, are constantly in the media, but now is not the time for you to be trying them out. If you have any questions or problems regarding diet, don't be tempted to take the well-meaning advice of a friend, who in all likelihood hasn't a clue about what is best for you. Your doctor will be happy to advise you on the foods you need, and the foods you don't; or he may want to refer you to a competent dietitian.

If you are concerned about whether or not you can resume normal sexual activity without detriment, you will be happy to learn that most people do who have suffered a myocardial infarction. Although you should avoid intercourse when you are over tired or under heavy emotional strain, your doctor will likely confirm that resuming normal sexual relations will be of benefit to you psychologically. (Avoid intercourse immediately after large meals, however.) Moderation is the keynote.

A great deal of research is presently being done on heart disease. As a result, the mass media are often bulging with the latest reports. It is important to remember that these reports are usually written by people uneducated in the medical field; consequently they are often misleading. Statistics may be weighted by the writer, or incomplete facts reported. Sometimes, too, an article is written based on outdated information; you may be led to false hopes of a new cure. Remember that you have a doctor in whom you have confidence and trust; don't hesitate to use him. It is his job to be available, and he is the best person to advise you of your treatment.

A prominent Toronto cardiologist suggests a simple walking programme for his cardiac patients. Because it is free and accessible, he feels that walking is also free of excuses for not exercising. He also points out that no special outfit or equipment is required, no membership dues collected, and since there are no watchers, it is free of competition as well. He usually suggests that, during the first week at home, his patients take small walks around the house. In the second week, he advises them to sit outside and get a little fresh air if the weather is not inclement. After that, this specialist suggests you begin your walking programme. Start by walking a distance of four or five houses, and increase your distance by one house per day, as long as you have no unpleasant symptoms, until you are walking one to two miles daily. Try timing yourself to the end of your walk. Repeat the same course daily; try to knock off a few seconds each day.

Because you must avoid cold or windy weather, it is suggested that you find an indoor shopping centre and do your walking there when it isn't too busy. If you live in an apartment, you may simply walk around the halls. Or you may want to do your walking in a school gym or church basement. Remember, in any case, if you notice the development of side effects, *stop what you are doing.*

There are three things you *must* avoid at all costs: (1) snow shovelling; (2) pushing a car; (3) house painting. Apart from that, a happy normal life can be yours again.

An Average Programme for First 3 Months after a Coronary Heart Attack

FIRST WEEK AT HOME – YOU ARE ALLOWED TO:

Go to the bathroom and shave, shower or bathe in tepid water.

Have all meals at the table.

Watch TV, listen to the radio, read newspapers.

Be up and about the house (climb stairs slowly if you must)

Have visitors.

Have one drink of liquor at lunch and/or supper, as desired.

Eat small, frequent meals.

FIRST WEEK AT HOME – AVOID:

Smoking.

Constipation. (Take adequate fluids including juices; take prunes and figs. If necessary, take a mild stool softener, such as mineral oil, Metamucil, or Colace. Milk of magnesia [30 cc], cascara [8 cc] or other mild cathartics may be taken if needed.)

Excitement, stress, and fatigue. (Get 8 to 9 hours of sleep a night; take a nap every morning and afternoon.)

Large meals, gassy foods, spiced or greasy foods.

Sex relations.

SECOND WEEK AT HOME – YOU ARE NOW ALLOWED:

Greater activity at home with shorter rest periods. To assist in light duties around the house. Sedentary hobbies and games (with the avoidance of undue emotional stress). Essential business conferences, provided they are not too numerous, or protracted, or associated with tension.

THIRD AND FOURTH WEEKS AT HOME – YOU MAY NOW:

Go out-of-doors in good weather.

Walk one block and increase daily as tolerated so that you may be walking 4 blocks by the end of this period.

Climb stairs; start with half a flight and gradually increase to 1 or 2 flights, if necessary.

THIRD AND FOURTH WEEKS AT HOME – AVOID:

Cold or windy weather.

Walking uphill.

Fatigue, exhaustion, emotional stress.

Walking or exertion immediately after eating.

Carrying heavy packages.

FIFTH THROUGH EIGHTH WEEK AT HOME –
YOU MAY NOW:

Resume sex activities in moderation.

Resume normal social activities. (Avoid fatigue and emotional strain.)

Return to work part-time after consulting your physician. (The exact time will be governed by the type of work and the progress of your recovery).

FIFTH THROUGH EIGHTH WEEK AT HOME –
AVOID:

Overeating.
Gain in weight.
Fatigue, tension.
Exhaustion.
All sports.

TOWARD THE END OF THIS PERIOD CONSULT YOUR PHYSICIAN ABOUT THE FOLLOWING:

A. Resumption of work.   B. Driving a car.   C. Participation in recreational activities.

TWELVE WEEKS AFTER HEART ATTACK – YOU MAY:

Resume all activities that you performed prior to your heart attack.

TWELVE WEEKS AFTER HEART ATTACK – AVOID:

Competitive sports. Smoking
Prolonged or excessive working hours.

Body reconditioning through exercise may contribute to the over-all improvement of the convalescence. (Discuss with your doctor.) Notify your physician in case of:

1. Sudden onset of chest pain.
2. Marked shortness of breath.
3. Palpitations (either rapid heart action or skipped beats).
4. Sudden weight gain (3 lbs in two days or 5 lbs in any one week).

5. Swelling of the feet.
6. Inability to lie flat in bed (due to shortness of breath, coughing or wheezing).
7. Extreme fatigue or profuse sweating.
8. Fainting spells.
9. Any other unusual symptom.

Note: Vague aches and pains in the chest are very common after a heart attack and are usually not significant. Inability to draw a deep breath and frequent yawning episodes are common and also have no serious connotations.

This chart adapted from *Treatment of Heart Disease in the Adult* by Rubin, Gross and Arbeit, 2nd edition, Lea & Febiger, Philadelphia, 1972.

More About Penguins and Pelicans

Penguinews, which appears every month, contains details of all the new books issued by Penguins as they are published. From time to time it is supplemented by our stocklist, which includes around 5,000 titles.

A specimen copy of *Penguinews* will be sent to you free on request. Please write to Dept EP, Penguin Books Ltd, Harmondsworth, Middlesex, for your copy.

In the U.S.A.: For a complete list of books available from Penguins in the United States write to Dept CS, Penguin Books, 625 Madison Avenue, New York, New York 10022.

In Canada: For a complete list of books available from Penguins in Canada write to Penguin Books Canada Ltd, 2801 John Street, Markham, Ontario L3R 1B4.